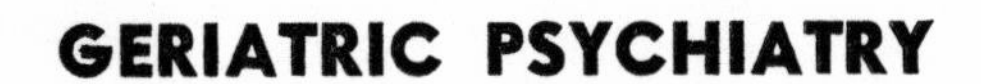

GERIATRIC PSYCHIATRY

GERIATRIC PSYCHIATRY

By

KURT WOLFF, M.D.

Associate Chief of Staff

for

Research and Education
Veterans Administration Hospital
Coatesville, Pennsylvania

and

Associate in Psychiatry
The University of Pennsylvania Medical School

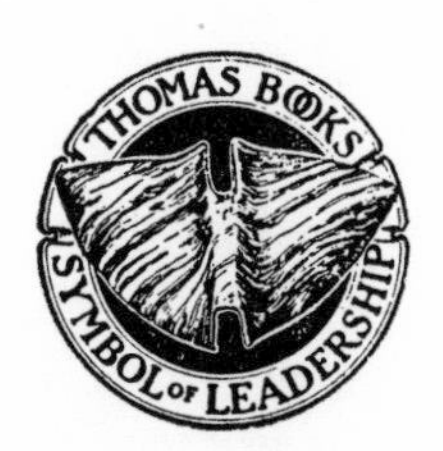

CHARLES C THOMAS · PUBLISHER
Springfield · Illinois · U.S.A.

Published and Distributed Throughout the World by
CHARLES C THOMAS • PUBLISHER
BANNERSTONE HOUSE
301-327 East Lawrence Avenue, Springfield, Illinois, U.S.A.

Library of Congress Catalog Card Number: 62-20596

With THOMAS BOOKS careful attention is given to all details of manufacturing and design. It is the Publisher's desire to present books that are satisfactory as to their physical qualities and artistic possibilities and appropriate for their particular use. THOMAS BOOKS will be true to those laws of quality that assure a good name and good will.

Printed in the United States of America

To

Senior Citizens All Over
the World

INTRODUCTION

During the last seven years the progress of psychiatry has been great; the development of new methods of treatment, revolutionary. Every year we are learning more about the causes of "mental sickness" in emotionally disturbed children, in mental deficiency, and in schizophrenia. A coordinated approach involving biological research methods, sociological approaches and psychodynamic viewpoints is gaining more and more followers in the medical world. The excellent books of Bellak (10) and of Jackson (83) give proof of this important change. In Geriatrics, however, such a coordinated and integrated approach is still a dream of the future. Biologically oriented gerontologists believe only in statistically proven facts. Sociologists frequently come to contradictory results but are nevertheless making great progress in studying the environmental factors involved in the process of Aging. The medical world remains skeptical about the possibilities of treating the geriatric patient but recognizes the urgency of the problem. The number of psychiatrists interested in treating the emotionally disturbed geriatric patients continues to be very small. However, the very few psychiatrists working on this problem have established the fact that the elderly "mental patient" is treatable by psychiatric methods when handled with empathy and patience. The spiritual reward in helping such "hopeless" cases is great indeed.

This book is written to stimulate further research in Geriatric Psychiatry, to point out the gravity and importance of the problem of the elderly "mental" patient, and to indicate some possibilities of treatment worthy of further investigation and exploration. It is not to be considered a textbook of Geriatrics. It is not a complete and final study of Geriatric Psychiatry but only a beginning. However, it is the fruit of many years of experience and study of treatment methods for geriatric patients in psychiatric institutions.

ACKNOWLEDGMENTS

I AM indebted and deeply grateful to: John A. Doering, M.D., Hospital Director, and Marcus P. Rosenblum, M.D., Chief of Staff, of the Veterans Administration Hospital, Coatesville (Pa.), for their encouragement and great interest in geriatric research; to Jerrold Bonn, M.D., Philadelphia; to David Cohen, Ph.D., Chief, Psychology Service, VA Hospital, Coatesville (Pa.); to Albert E. Scheflen, M.D., Associate Professor of Psychiatry, Temple University, Philadelphia, for reading the manuscript and giving invaluable advice; and finally to Miss Virginia Domblesky of the VA Hospital, Coatesville, for the secretarial assistance.

KURT WOLFF, M.D.

CONTENTS

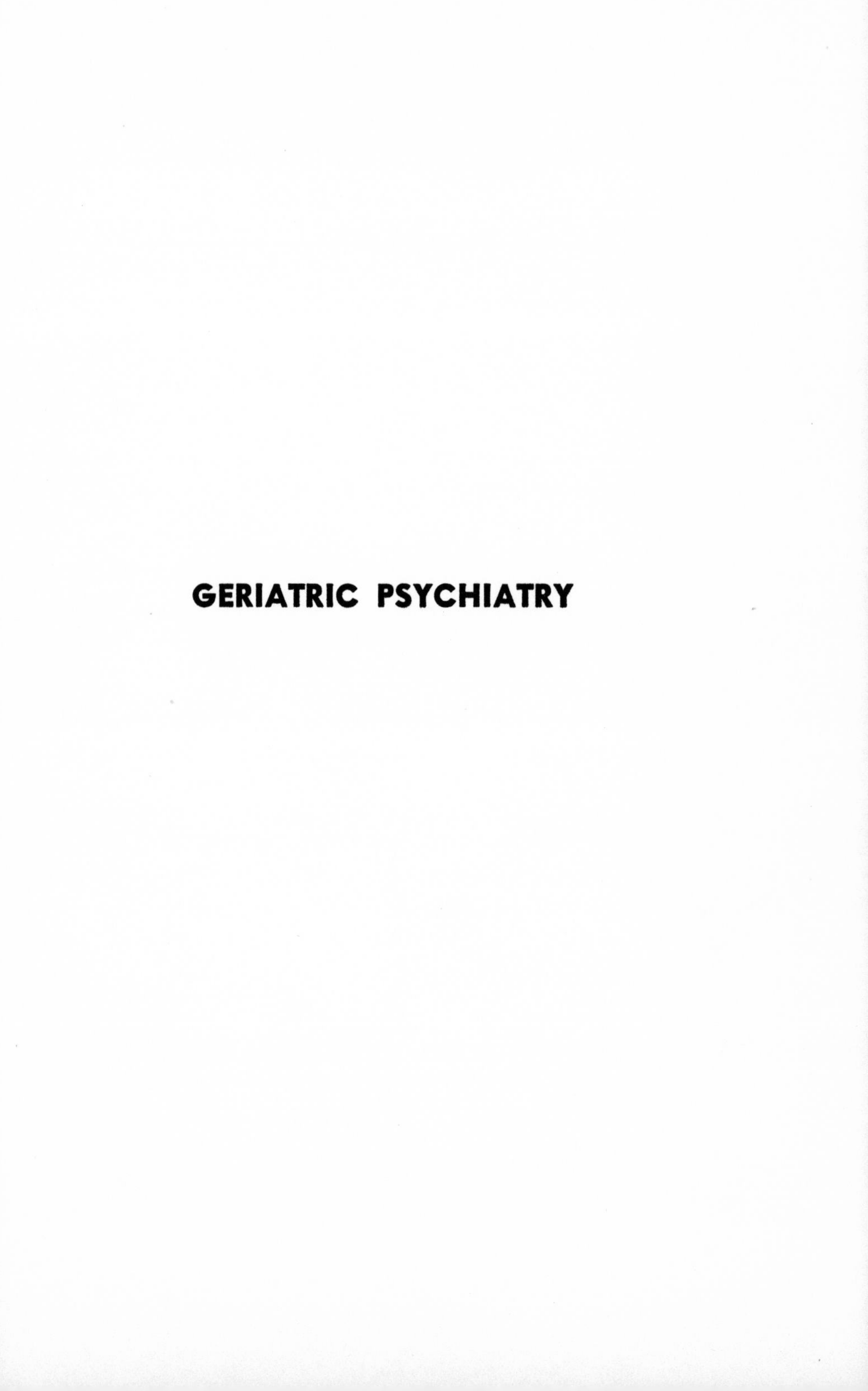

GERIATRIC PSYCHIATRY

1

THE GERIATRIC PATIENT— A NATIONAL AND INTERNATIONAL PROBLEM

THE PERCENTAGE of the total population of the United States 65 years of age and over has increased from 4% in 1900 to 8.1% in 1950. It is expected to increase to 10% by 1970. In 1953, there were 13,325,000 persons 65 years of age and over in the United States. The number is increasing at the rate of about 350,000 a year. At present we have about 16 million people over the age of 65. This number, according to N. W. Shock (139), will probably increase to 32 million in the next 40 years. H. D. Sheldon (135) states that the proportion of older persons (defined either as persons 65 and over, or 60 and over) nearly doubled in the 50-year period from 1900 to 1950. A critical review of statistics of elderly persons in the United States and throughout the world, made by Sheldon, revealed that the "underdeveloped countries" are the countries with "young populations," whereas the countries with "older populations" are the industrialized countries of Western Europe and their offshoots in other parts of the world. While Brazil, Egypt and Ceylon, for instance, have a relatively greater percentage of younger population, France, Germany, Great Britain and the United States count a relatively greater percentage of older people.

H. F. Page (123), in an interesting study on the "Medical Aspects of the Health Care Needs of the Elderly Patient," reports that the average length of life about 2000 years ago (in Rome) was 22 years; in the Middle Ages (in Great Britain) 33 years; in 1900 in the United States, 49.2 years; in 1946 in the United States, 66.7 years. The life expectancy for males in the United States is about 67 years; for females, almost 73 years.

This steadily increasing number of persons over 65 years of age has created a special problem for our hospitals. According to N. W. Shock (139), people over 65 spend 2½ times as many days in hospitals as those under 65. They comprise almost one-third of the hospitalized population. For psychiatric hospitals this higher percentage of elderly persons, augmented every year, has become of the greatest importance.

From 1936 to 1951, the number of persons 65 years and over in the population increased 57.5%. During the same period, according to Lawrence Kolb (96), the number of first admissions of persons 65 and over to state mental hospitals increased 95.3%. J. Donnelly reports that the number of patients admitted to state hospitals in the United States with the diagnosis of Chronic Brain Syndrome associated with Senility or Cerebral Arteriosclerosis, already approaches the number of patients admitted with the diagnosis of Schizophrenia. Bettag and his Associates (12) made the observation that as of January 1, 1955, nearly one-third of all patients in Illinois state mental hospitals were 65 years and older. Of these, approximately one-half were admitted while still under 65 and approximately one-half were admitted after reaching the age of 65. According to these authors, only one patient in five in these groups will be discharged from the Illinois state hospitals alive. The other four will end their days under state care. Bettag and his Associates predicted that in the year 2000, 67% of the patients in state hospitals and 30.2% of the national population will be over 65.

Generally speaking during 1960 and 1961, about 30% of all new admissions to state psychiatric institutions were 60 years of age and over. In most psychiatric state institutions throughout the United States, at the present time, more than 45% of the patients are over 60 years of age.

According to statistics of the Federal Council on Aging (53), Washington, D. C., in 1959 there were 22,666,000 veterans of World Wars I and II in civil life. By 1960, veterans of World War I 65 years of age or over numbered about 1,688,000. In 1964 it is estimated that 2,106,000 World War I veterans will be in this age bracket. The number of patients in VA hospitals increases with age: in the age group 55 to 64, 55.2% of the veterans are under VA care; when veterans reach the age of 65 or over, about 58.6% are treated by the Veterans Administration. According to our Census (January 1962) at Coatesville VA Hospital, 37.5% of our patients were veterans of the First World War and over 60 years of age. Most of our psychiatric patients in this age group are chronic schizophrenics, while the number of acute or chronic brain syndromes is relatively small. We expect an increase in our elderly psychiatric, neurologic and medical patient population as time goes on.

According to E. L. Bortz (16), the percentage of the population of the United States over 65 will continue to grow and life expectancy rates will expand to the point that persons who reach maturity can, with some confidence, anticipate living into their 70s, 80s or 90s. By 1970, the number of persons in the United States over 65 years of age will probably number in the vicinity of 22,000,000. In the same period, the number of persons over 45 will increase to about 65,000,000, or roughly half the entire adult population. Of these, women over 45 will probably outnumber men by 6,000,000 and women over 65 will exceed men in the same age bracket by about 3,000,000. Finally, if we are able to control many more common disorders and diseases, an even greater expansion of the life span of our population in the U.S.A. can be expected.

To the same degree, the same increase of life expctancy can be predicted for all countries of the world with the development of adequate public hygiene programs and increasing industrialization. These "underdeveloped" countries who continue with unimproved hygienic methods, with serious lack of physicians and hospitals to control infectious diseases, and with a population suffering from malnutrition, will continue to show a relatively high mortality rate.

A recent publication from Australia, however, brings us some interesting material of the concern of the medical profession even in this relatively young country in regard to the problem of the aging population. Already about 10% of the population in Australia is over 65 and nearly 30% of these are chronic patients in general or psychiatric hospitals. Under the guidance of E. C. Dax (44), Chairman, Mental Hygiene Authority, Victoria, an intensive program for the elderly patient with emotional disturbances is emphasized. Dax believes that "there are great possibilities to come from the better study of geriatric psychiatry, with interest in research and prevention of illness in the avoidance of mental disturbances." According to this scientist, there is still much to be learned about the proper accommodation and arrangements for these cases if this disturbance does occur. Dax recommends as a first step, the treatment of the geriatric patients in their own homes. He feels that there is a good chance of doing this with modern drugs. If these fail, there is still a good prognosis for many, according to Dax, if they are adequately treated by well-trained personnel with techniques which are active, constructive and helpful. It is as unwise to think of the mentally disturbed geriatric patient as senile as to think of the mental hospital as a place for custodial and terminal care.

Alan Stoller (144), Chief Clinical Officer, Mental Hygiene Authority, Victoria, points out that there are a large number of elderly people in Australia whose mental health needs are not being adequately met. Mental illness is considered by Stoller as a sign of unsuccessful aging and is involved in all aspects of illness and maladjustment among the aged. According to Stoller, our progressive industrialization and urbanization leads to a high value being placed on the younger elements in our society. There is, in Australia, an urgent need to reorient the community in general, the professional workers who work with the aged, as well as the aging popuation itself, toward this fact. These facts therefore justify the development of a general community program which will provide education of the mental health needs of older people.

In Europe, especially in Great Britain, France, West Germany, Sweden, Norway, Denmark, the Netherlands and Belgium, where the increase of the aging population is very similar to that of the United States, programs in support of the aged have been adapted to meet the customs, practices and social characteristics of the particular country. Outstanding members of the U. S. Veterans Administration (31) medical staff visited these countries in the summer of 1960 and wrote an extensive report about their findings and observations in regard to treatment facilities and methods in these West-European countries. Caring for the aged in Western Europe is no longer looked upon as a matter of charity but as a requirement of social justice. The aged are considered to be full and active members of society. The general philosophy behind European treatment methods implies that the aged should be enabled to live independently and to take care of themselves as long as possible. They are treated therefore, preferably in their own homes. Only when home care becomes too risky, too difficult, or too expensive, are they transferred to an institution. Of special value is the progressive approach of the Geriatric Unit at the Cowley Road Hospital, Oxford, Great Britain, under the leadership of L. Z. Cosin. (37, 38)

Cosin recommends a close cooperation of medical in- and outpatient treatment for geriatric patients and emphasizes the need to maintain the independence of the older person in the community while sharing responsibility with the family and the community for those patients who are more frail. In Oxford, through the combined effort and close cooperation of the general practitioner, community services, domiciliary visiting, outpatient departments, the day hospitals, the "hostels" and the geriatric hospital staff, results are obtained which are far superior to anything, I believe, we are able to show to the world in the United States at the present time. Although many millions of dollars are spent every year for gerontological research, and new and original treatment methods are studied in many university clinics, research centers, VA hospitals, general hospitals and state mental institutions, geriatric psychiatry is still very much neglected in present-day United States and is in need of urgent consideration.

2

DEFINITION OF THE GERIATRIC PATIENT

Gerontologists agree that chronological age is related to but not identical with "aging." According to J. E. Birren (13), young and old men differ in many behavioral and biological characteristics; however, man and lower organisms have determinate life spans and show systemic changes with advancing chronological age. Birren advocates dropping the term "aging" eventually and replacing it with terms like "longevity," "senescence" or "antiquation." He further emphasizes differences among "biological age," "psychological age" and "social age" and believes that these differences demand specific consideration. To him, "biological age" is correlated with chronological age, but also independent of it to some extent; "physiological age" is considered in relation to mortality rates; "psychological age" is defined as the sum of achievements and potentials of an individual; while "social age" refers to acquired social status and habits, to the individual's filling the many social roles or expectancies of a person of his age in his culture and social group. The criterion of biological age is length of life; of psychological age, the capacity of adaptation. The criteria of social age are social output and performance. Birren points out that social role performance may improve with age, whereas the adaptive capacity of the individual may decline.

R. G. Kuhlen (98) argues that the definition of aging should include not merely chronological age but also the more individual and personal variables. This gerontologist demonstrates the fruitfulness of studying aging within the framework of a more general theory and of a better conceptualization of increased chronological age. According to Kuhlen, the degree to which the various phases of life (various age periods) offer basic gratifications or pose serious threats and thus influence adjustment depends upon such variables as: the meaning of life and of aging to the individual; the role he occupies at a given age rather than his chronological age; his general "style of life" and personality make-up (rigidity—flexibility); situational factors that may pose environmental stresses; and personal factors (capacities) which not only may be threatening in their own right but also may reduce the individual's ability to cope successfully with his environment and to achieve gratifications in usual ways and intensities.

E. L. Bortz (17), too, believes that chronological age should not be considered as the principal measure of longevity. He states that this is a particularly inadequate concept since the passage of time affects people in different ways. Aging begins with the genetic endowment. The rate of aging varies with each individual and is affected in many ways by environmental influences for better or for worse. Different parts of the body age at different rates. There are old persons in their thirties and young ones in their nineties. It is possible to double the life span of lower animals. It is also possible in the human, providing the individual himself is sufficiently motivated to redirect habits of personal hygiene.

Much attention has been given to the role, in aging, of the atrophy of cells—especially in the brain cortex—and to the atrophy of organ system—especially the musculature. A clear explanation in regard to the cause and origin of these specific atrophies is still to be set forth. N. W. Shock (138, 140) believes that a large proportion of muscular atrophy is due to disuse. He bases this belief on observations of athletes who do not show atrophy of their muscle cells due to continuous exercise. Shock emphasizes the factor of motivation. While we know much about physical conditioning and athletic performance in younger persons, we are not sure whether middle-aged people can restore many of their functional capacities by progressive exercise. According to Shock, the answer can be found only by studying groups of sedentary middle-aged persons motivated to carry through a series of long-term experiments of this kind. Until this is systematically studied, the exact amount of impairment and cellular loss due to atrophy of disuse will remain unknown.

In contrast to Shock, H. Selye (134) gives greater importance to the factor of "wear and tear." According to Selye, there is a great difference between physiological and chronologic age. One person can be much more senile in body and mind, and much closer to the grave, at forty years than another person at sixty years. Selye states that true age depends largely on the rate of wear and tear, on the speed of self-consumption. To him, life is essentially a process which gradually spends the given amount of "adaptation energy" that we inherited from our parents. Vitality is like a special kind of bank account which you can use up by withdrawals but cannot increase by deposits. The person's control over this most precious fortune is the rate at which withdrawals are made. The solution is evidently not to stop withdrawing, for this would be death. Nor is it to withdraw just enough for survival, for this would permit only a vegetative life—worse than death. The intelligent thing to do is to withdraw generously, but never expend wastefully. Selye explains furthermore that the belief of restoration by rest after exposure to very stressful activities is a false one. Experiments on animals have clearly shown that each exposure to stress leaves an indelible scar because the animals are using up reserves of adaptability which cannot be replaced. It is true, according to Selye, that immediately after some harassing experience, rest can restore us *almost* to the original level of fitness by eliminating acute fatigue. But the emphasis is on the word *almost.* Since we constantly go through periods of stress and rest during life, even a little deficit of adaptation energy every day adds up. It adds up to what we call aging.

E. J. Stieglitz (143) considers aging as part of living; it cannot be arrested without terminating life. It begins with conception and terminates only with death. Its course and consequences may be altered and perhaps retarded, but they cannot be stopped so long as life goes on. Aging, according to Stieglitz, may be defined as the dimension of time in the processes of living. It involves two processes which go on simultaneously from the beginning to the end: growth or evolution, and atrophy or involution. We see involutional phenomena in the embyro—the disappearance of embryonic clefts. In the newborn, the atrophy of the ductus arteriosus is identical with the obliterative arterial changes later in life. Growth continues throughout the life span. Use creates growth and disuse, atrophy. But although these two processes go on simultaneously throughout the life span, from birth until death, they progress asymmetrically. The most interesting and probably the most important factor of the biological process of aging is, according to Stieglitz, the fact that changes associated with aging are not uniform or symmetrical. Stieglitz believes that aging is both wearing out from use and, paradoxically, atrophy from disuse. The vigorous, active individual with compulsive tendencies is inclined to assume that we rust from disuse and so justifies his continued activity. On the other hand, the more introverted and passive individual would be inclined to become more easily fatigued by greater activities of his body and mind and would rationalize that we age faster due to exhaustion.

Both theories on aging point out important facts and are based on clinical and experimental observations. However, the factor of homeostasis* must be brought into the definition of aging, to be integrated into the function of use-disuse and stress. This is especially important if we consider aging as a biological, sociological and psychological phenomenon. The cells of the brain and of our musculature shrink definitely when we do not use them and keep them inactive. Our psychological assets and our social adaptive possibilities atrophy, too, when we remain in a passive non-alert attitude of mind and do not reach out for intellectual or social goals. The achievement of these is not possible without a certain degree of strain and compulsive activity. On the other hand, too much compulsion and overactivity without relaxation, without rest and periods of introspection and meditation will result in the antithesis of real creativity: rigid, tense, inflexible, over-

---

* The term "hemeostasis" has been introduced into physiology by W. B. Cannon and into psychiatry by Karl Menninger. It means an omnipresent tendency toward maintaining equilibrium and stability in the organism.

active attitude which will break like a cord when it is torn, and leave the person fatigued, exhausted, weak and feeling older. The right equilibrium of activity and rest, of stress and respose, of goal directed activity and introverted meditation (self-analysis), is the most suitable formula for staying young, vigorous and creative. This equilibrium, however, depends on highly individual factors.

There are individuals for whom a certain physical or emotional stress might fall "in a normal range," while for others the same activity is conducive to fatigue or, on the contrary, results in being too passive and without sufficient motivation and goal directed action. Aging is a highly individual phenomenon for which one specific formula cannot be applied for all people. Therefore, we must be satisfied to study the aging process on a more general level and then apply our findings on a highly individual basis. This is the problem of the "geriatric patient" who suffers because of getting older. His reaction to this process is a worthwhile study and should inspire all our therapeutic efforts when he becomes our patient.

There is no doubt that the geriatric patient, as has already been pointed out by Birren (13) in his definition of aging, represents a biological, sociological and psychological entity. Consequently, in therapy, we have to be aware that the geriatric patient and his successful treatment can and should be handled only by a coordinated approach which must involve the efforts of the psychiatrist, the internist and also the general practitioner who must apply his biological and psychological knowledge with judgment and common sense. Thus it is reasonable to me, before describing my own therapeutic experiences as a psychiatrist with geriatric patients in psychiatric institutions, to outline briefly the biological, sociological and psychological features to be taken into consideration when handling a geriatric patient, in the hope that it may lead to a better understanding and closer cooperation between the different disciplines of medicine.

3

THE COORDINATED APPROACH TO THE GERIATRIC PROBLEM

SINCE the geriatric patient represents a biologic, psychologic, and sociological unity, only a coordinated approach, taking into consideration all three aspects, will help us in solving the urgent and important problems he presents.

Great progress has been achieved during the last 10 years by research done exploring the biological aspect of geriatrics.

Himwich, H. E., and Himwich, W. A. (80), give much importance to the fact that after 40 years of age the basal metabolic rate or the oxygen consumption of the entire body gradually falls, with a more rapid rate decrease after 80 years of age. The Himwiches have observed a gradual increase of water in the cerebral cortex at the expense of solid elements in old age, that metabolism decreases and the brain appears to shrink. They found that both the white and the gray matter of the cerebral cortex show an accumulation of moisture in old age and believe that the gradual increase of water at the expense of solid elements, along with morphological alterations, may represent the basis for mental impairment of the elderly. Buerger (20) made extensive studies in regard to chemical changes of the brain in elderly persons. He showed that the amount of proteins, and especially the values of glutamic acid, in the brain tissue diminish. The Himwiches suggest that, generally, in old age, compounds containing nitrogen and phosphorus decrease in the brain, while sulfur compounds increase at the age of 90.

Kety (91, 92) believes that the loss of neurons, the progressive deterioration of certain essential cellular components and the decrease in neuronal interconnections and interactions are important factors in the process of aging. Kety maintains that the fall in the circulation and oxygen supply for the brain from childhood to old age is basic to all other chemical, biological and functional changes.

Shock (138) confirms the importance of the decreased basal metabolism in old persons. For Shock, the reduction in total metabolism is simply a reflection of the reduced number of metabolizing units (cells) present in the organism of the elderly person.

Lansing (99) points out that the older individual is prone to accumulate fat, has reduced physical capacities, deteriorated vision and suffers from a lack of adaptability to environmental changes. He believes that calcium, in some way, plays an important role in establishing the aging process because calcium lowers cells' permeability.

Gerard (63) relates the phenomena of aging especially to the nervous system. According to Gerard, neurons decrease in size and number, the metabolic rate slows down, the cells contain more slag and decay and there is an accumulation of calcium which slows the function of the cells. In this way, growth becomes impossible. Aging, therefore, according to Gerard, is a failure of regenerative, reconstructive and rejuvenative processes.

Freeman (59) has studied the influence of the endocrines on the aging body and observed that while there may be a decrease of ACTH production with age, the only constant endocrine alteration characteristic of old age is gonadal failure.

C. F. Geschickter (66) comes to the conclusion that aging may be due to a gradually increasing discrepancy between the demands of specialization by the tissues and the available metabolic support. Since most tissues are dependent upon their blood supply for nourishment, and since natural aging is a slow and progressive decline of function, these regressive changes in the tissue are in general correlated with changes in the blood supply. If diminution of the blood supply proceeds too rapidly, the tissue will undergo a form of atrophy, which may be classed as accelerated aging. On the other hand, if damage to the tissue exceeds that to the blood supply, resolution, organization and fibrotic repair or regeneration will replace the aging process. Natural aging, therefore, presupposes a certain degree of correlation between parenchymal and vascular changes, with the rate and amount of tissue lost being roughly proportional to the declining vascular status of the individual organ affected.

Geschickter is of the opinion that a number of metabolic factors can accelerate the aging process. The most readily demonstrable are those arising from exogenous deprivation, such as starvation, low protein intake, and lack of fat or lack of vitamin B complex absorption in the bowel. Endogenous disturbances of the metabolism are more numerous and more intricate in bringing about accelerated aging. The most universal endogenous metabolic factor is interference with the vascular supply. Since we have found acceleration of the aging processes in joints in subjects of advanced renal disease, it is probable, according to Geschickter, that vascular disturbance operates both through the production of hypoxia and the diminished removal of metabolic waste products.

Barnes, Busse and co-workers (9) have made special studies on brain wave changes in elderly persons and found a slowing of the alpha rhythm in normally functioning elderly persons and an even greater slowing associated with psychologic decline. In addition, a special focal disturbance has been found in "normal" subjects over the age of 60, as well as in subjects suffering from organic brain disease. In 80% of the cases, these dysrhythmias are located in the left temporal area, most often in the anterior temporal region.

The result of these biological studies on aging can be summarized in the following findings. Aging produces:

1. An increase in connective tissues in the organism.
2. A gradual loss of elastic properties of connective tissue.
3. Disappearance of cellular elements in the Nervous System.
4. A reduction of the number of normally functioning cells.
5. An increased amount of fat.
6. A decrease in oxygen utilization.
7. A decrease in the cardiac output at rest, particularly in the cerebral blood flow.
8. A decrease in the maximal breathing capacity of the lungs.
9. A decrease in muscle strength.

10. A lowered hormonal output, especially by the gonads and the adrenal glands.
11. A gradual increase of water at the expense of solid elements.

Many biologists have given thought to the higher incidence of arteriosclerosis in populations where the fat content of the diet is high. This theory has led to the recommendation of reduction of fat in the diet as protection against arteriosclerosis. It seems, however, that saturated fats from animal sources play a greater role than unsaturated fats from vegetables, in the development of arteriosclerosis. According to statistics given by insurance companies, over-weight in adults definitely reduces life expectancy. Inadequate intake of proteins, minerals and vitamins also appears to play an important role in reducing our life span. Old people, apparently, are more prone to consume a higher amount of carbohydrates, due, perhaps, to poor dentition.

The sociological factors to be considered in connection with the geriatric problem derive from stresses connected with the elderly person's occupation, environment, family and community. These stresses frequently are related to a disturbed emotional equilibrium. Among these sociological factors of great influence on the aging process, the factor of retirement is perhaps the most important one.

Retirement indeed is, according to my own experience, the most frequent precipitating factor causing emotional upsets in elderly people which may lead to hospitalization. When older persons do not have hobbies and interests, developed in earlier years, which are able to occupy their time and thus their minds after retirement, they are unable to relax and to enjoy life. Too much leisure makes them feel useless and superfluous, causes them to concentrate their interest on their physical status, and gives origin to many psychosomatic complaints and to depressions. Retirement often causes a severe loss of self-esteem. To lose one's goal in life means, for many old persons, the end of all their hopes and of life itself. Many old people have for years held their mind and body together by compulsive work. They simply are not used to relaxation. Not knowing what recreation means, they have in later life a complete breakdown of their physical and mental health, accompanied by sudden and severe confusion and disorganization. They are really "lost" in the true and symbolic sense of the word.

Elderly persons, therefore, must not only retire from something, but must have something to retire to. To find suitable hobbies and interests for them, to make them relax and be less anxious, to help them to "recreate" a new life is indeed one of the most important goals of our preventive treatment program.

In contrast to these observations (confirmed by many psychiatrists), E. Cumming, L. R. Dean, D. S. Newell and J. McCaffrey (41) consider aging as a disengaging process leading to a "disengaged state." These researchers have done an extensive study in Kansas City (the Kansas City Study of Adult Life, a project of the Committee on Human Development of the University of Chicago) on 211 healthy elderly persons between the ages of 50 and 70. They believe that elderly individuals withdraw from our social system rather than being deserted by others. According to Cummings and co-workers, this disengagement begins during the sixth decade of their life and reflects a withdrawal of "object cathexis" and a beginning of anticipatory socialization to the aged state. Interactions with members of the younger age group are constricted and the number of hours of each day spent in the company of others is reduced. The result of this "disengaging" process is a more self-centered style of behavior among the ambulatory aged.

There is some truth to the observation that elderly individuals frequently feel the necessity to be "left alone," that they become less social minded and more interested in their own emotional, spiritual and intellectual life, and that they frequently consume considerable time in thinking of their bodily ailments. However, they almost invariably feel ambivalent about their solitude. They realize that many activities of young people are undesirable for them and out of their domain. The majority of elderly citizens have less interest in the parties, dances, sports, technical interests, economical-political problems and nightly amusements so important for the younger generation. They are aware that they are in need of more sleep, of greater periods of rest and relaxation than younger people. They nonetheless resent being excluded from the younger generation's plans and interests on very many occasions, to be left more or less completely to their own devices. Although older persons withdraw at times voluntarily from many attitudes, customs and activities of younger people, they so frequently do so with resentment and disappointment, and stay in lonesome, unhappy seclusion. Their wish to encounter younger people "half way" and to find some common goal and interest, has often been rejected. A great number of elderly citizens do not want to intrude into the life of younger people due to their lack of understanding of the needs of the other generations, and also because of their fear of feeling unwanted. Many old people sometimes desperately reach out to meet younger people but without success due to misunderstanding and lack of empathy on both sides.

The second factor of very great influence on the emotional and physical health of our aged, is our cultural attitude toward them. Our century is the "century of youth." We are all directed toward social and economical goals, are driven by an unresistable force to achieve them. We live in a world of continuous competition and therefore we have to work compulsively and strenuously to improve our social position and maintain it. We live in continuous anxiety. We decide that "time is money." We are overburdened with work, have no time for recreation, for relaxation, and, sometimes, not even for sleep. We lose the connection with the beauty of the natural world and with the rhythm of life. Music, art, literature, for us, are considered a "waste of time." We fail to find relaxation in our family life, not even in love. Emotionally detached sexuality frequently has taken the place of true love, and the responsibilities of our family life make us worry day and night. We live without imagination, without play, without fantasy, without romance. We sometimes lose the feeling of being human beings and do things mechanically and without interest. Then, as the end of our life comes nearer to us, we are exhausted and have the feeling we have not really lived at all. In such a world of tension, of compulsion, of work and of competition, elderly people are considered a burden. They know it, they feel it, they see and hear it and are unhappy and dejected. Elderly people can't compete with this modern trend any more, and they are unable to change it. We, however, can and should do something about it.

Especially appropriate in this connection is Linden's paper, "Relationship Between Social Attitudes Toward Aging and the Delinquencies of Youth." (104) He points out the connection between our lack of respect toward the elderly person and indeed our attitudes of rejection, intolerance, impatience, hostility and annoyance with the elderly parents or grandparents and the increase of juvenile delinquency. Children who can't identify with father or grandfather, who consider elderly parents useless and burdensome, who laugh about Senior Citizens, who grow up without parental support and without ethical judgment, are frequently in a state of rebellion. A culture where life experience and wisdom are held in no esteem, where parents and grandparents are not felt to be examples of goodness and personal worthiness, where authority is rebelled against because it is not considered important, must create simultaneously an atmosphere of freedom without limits, of wanting without boundaries, and of egocentricity. When the child does not learn to look upon the elderly as an object of respect, then the door is open for rebellion and disobedience. Police control never can substitute for parental support. Punitive measures will never be as effective as the parents' love and understanding. Linden concludes that our own cultural attitude is therefore partially to blame for the increasing delinquency of our children.

The third factor to consider is the feeling of economic insecurity from which so many old folks suffer. Old people have to live protected from the most urgent needs of our daily life. Public welfare helps, we know, when need arises, but this help should be given willingly and effectively so as not to cause an emotional blow and severe loss of self-esteem. Special housing projects, hospitals for the chronically sick, rehabilitation and recreation centers have to be built. Only in this way can we prevent many emotional and physical sicknesses of elderly persons. The accent should, however, never be on welfare but on rehabilitation. Most elderly persons can still do useful and meaningful work if they find understanding for their problems. They might work more slowly and finish a task far later than a young person would, but they are often able to work with great exactness. In Switzerland, for instance, many watchmakers are older people because of their greater experience and patience. In the U.S.A., to a limited degree, we are using the skill of elderly persons as furmakers, tailors and even as machinists. There are many examples of great contributions by the elderly in politics, in art, in philosophy, and in science. The achievements of Michelangelo, Churchill, Gandhi, Toscanini, Einstein, Albert Schweitzer, and "Grandma" Moses immediately come to mind. These are people who, in spite of their old age, have been able to create things of which all humanity is very proud. We do not need to take a pessimistic attitude in regard to elderly persons. They do not have to regress, to deteriorate, to become useless, or to be considered superfluous. They can offer something younger persons do not possess: wisdom, patience and life experience which should and can be utilized for the benefit of all of us.

The emotional needs of the elderly person have been described recently by a number of outstanding physicians and psychiatrists. It has been stated that the cause of many of the mental breakdowns in later life can be found in experiences during childhood and adolescence. We know that these early experiences play an important part in the origin of schizophrenia and manic depressive psychosis. Now we recognize that disturbances like involutional psychosis and senile dementia also have their roots in childhood experiences. Grotjahn (73) has pointed out that the extreme restlessness which we sometimes find in geriatric patients can be due to castration fear, from which they have suffered all their lives. I was able, by sodium amytal interviews, to confirm this idea. I frequently found a close connection between the fear of death and castration anxiety, since death was felt to be the final castration.

The irritability of older psychotics often has its source in their inability to cope with the environment as well as in physical decline. Apathy in elderly persons can be considered as an outcome of the detachment of the individual from painful memories and events of his life. Kaplan (86) states that one of the effects of losing friends and relatives is to give the older person not only a feeling of being alone in the world but also a feeling that, without social ties, he is unprotected and insecure. Of different opinion is Overholzer (122) who suggests that our attitude of overprotection of our old people results in personality change and that we should be careful not to accelerate, in older people, their entrance into a condition of dependent helplessness. Loss of independent activity frequently produces an emotional crisis. Retirement, for instance, gives more opportunity for introspection, for self-evaluation, for the development of delusional ideas and for regrets. Older men tend to be more seclusive and withdrawn than older women and are more inclined to cerebral arteriosclerosis, while women suffer more from senile dementia.

The problem of becoming aware of being old has been studied by Jones (86) and others. Subjects have been asked how and when they first noticed they were growing old. Jones found that, in most cases, the following precipitating symptoms were mentioned by his patients:

1. Breakdown of the locomotor apparatus.
2. Difficulties of a nervous kind.
3. Sense organ impairment.
4. Deterioration of the skin and the hair.
5. Increased tendency to fatigue.
6. Greater need for short periods of sleep during daytime.

It is well known that paranoid trends become more evident in senile persons especially if their personality traits have always been of a suspicious kind. Old people often feel unwanted, and this realization may be conducive to delusional ideas.

Frequently the content of the delusions centers around the idea of being robbed, of being poverty stricken, or of being poisoned. The tendency to commit suicide increases with the higher age group. The loss of loved ones or physical sickness with a poor prognosis may precipitate this tendency and always has to be given careful consideration. Criminal offenses generally decrease with old age, but sexual offenses, fraud, violation of the narcotic laws, arson and poisoning frequently bring older people to court and, afterwards, to mental institutions. Studies of the emotional needs of the elderly have been made by comparing their attitude with the attitude of the child. The child has unlimited energy, great ambition and psychic elasticity which helps to keep him from being hurt, and he reaches out for the future. The aged person finds his supply of energy diminishing. He fears the future, blinds himself to reality, and finds himself in a continuous state of disillusionment.

Meerloo (114) defines the geriatric patient as one who does not and cannot accept the reality of being mortal. He considers old age as a traumatic neurosis with continuing trauma. The old person becomes more self-absorbed and tests his vital functions continuously. It has been thought that diminishing of heart function symbolizes loss of love. Busse (24) has made the observation that hypochondriasis is more prevalent in the older than in the younger generation. Due to their special emotional and physical handicaps, elderly individuals are using hypochondriac complaints frequently to excuse their failures and shortcomings. In this way the older individual is able to maintain self-respect and to decrease his guilt feelings over his not being a success and his failure to achieve. According to Busse, overconcern with health is a defense against anxiety in the aged person by which he is soliciting sympathy, forgiveness and help. Busse found this defense especially difficult to treat.

I have observed that many geriatric patients have distinctly ambivalent feelings toward life and death. They often want to die, believing they have nothing to live for. They wish for cessation of their physical and mental preoccupations, but, when they feel the hour of death to be near, they become disturbed and afraid. They cling to others and want them near at all times. They especially fear the dark and request that the light be kept on all night. They may turn more toward religion, go to church often, confess themselves, and ask that their sins be forgiven. Religion gives them emotional support and tends to relieve them from the fear that everything will soon come to an end.

The intellectual assets and liabilities in old people, as contrasted to young adults, were studied by Miles (119) at Stanford University. He found that imagination seems to be ageless, and that verbal associations, interpretation of meaning, and recognition of relationships show less tendency to decline with age than do speed, organization, recall of unfamiliar material and difficult logical procedures. The total intelligence quotient scores show a progressive decline with advancing age. Wechsler (148) points out that the curves show a parallelism between loss of brain weight and decline of ability with age. Gitelson and Gilbert (67, 68), however, believe that motivation to keep healthy, mentally and physically, is a very important factor guarding against intellectual decline.

Birren (14) made special studies regarding changes in sensation, perception and learning and observed that with advancing age there is an increased latency in all voluntary responses. The older organism seems to require additional time to integrate or perceive information from the environment and to "program" the appropriate response. Longer response latencies appear to have their greatest consequence in complex or serial tasks. The inference is drawn that the capacity of the central nervous system to integrate complex activity is limited. However, the high redundancy inherent in our verbal and social skills tends to mask the appearance of age changes in the central nervous system. Generalizing, according to Birren, has to be avoided.

So much about the biological, the sociological and the emotional aspects of aging. The gap in our understanding of this so interesting and important problem is obvious. Even more important, however, is the fact that more physicians now recognize the enormity of the problem and are working to solve the manifold multidisciplinary questions which it poses.

4

THE SCREENING OF THE GERIATRIC PATIENT PRIOR TO ADMISSION TO A PSYCHIATRIC INSTITUTION AND TREATMENT ON AN OUTPATIENT BASIS

THE APPLICATIONS for admission of geriatric patients to a psychiatric institution are becoming more and more frequent. Many state mental hospitals are overcrowded with patients and the number of elderly patients asking for hospitalization increases yearly. They are brought to the hospital at times already committed by a court order. The hospital physician not admitting these would be exposed to punishment by law for not obeying a court order and not admitting a patient even though he disagrees with the commitment order and believes that commitment to a psychiatric institution with consequent loss of civil rights of the patient is not necessary.

More often, however, patients are brought to the psychiatric hospital on a voluntary basis, or, in some states, for a 90-day observation and treatment period. In many such cases, patients could be evaluated on an outpatient basis by a competent psychiatrist and treated as outpatients, so that hospitalization might be avoided.

When a patient is brought to the mental institution for a 90-day observation and treatment period, this amount of time can be significantly shortened if the psychiatric staff is convinced that only a few days of hospitalization are needed for the evaluation of the patient and that the patient can be treated without hospitalization.

Some superintendents of overcrowded state mental institutions are well aware that there is a great number of geriatric patients admitted for hospitalization who do not need it. The psychiatrist examining the papers at the time of admission—or prior to it—finds sometimes that the mental condition of the patient has been described as confused, threatening or delusional, and that the diagnosis of schizophrenic reaction has been given, without sufficient substantiation. On the first and subsequent psychiatric examination at the psychiatric hospital, the diagnosis of the family physician cannot be confirmed. The question should be immediately asked as to why the patient had been found in need of urgent hospitalization. Does he really need to be hospitalized at all?

For this reason, I found it necessary to re-examine applications of geriatric patients to a state mental hospital and have done a study on 105 elderly patients. The results were very revealing. There was clearly an exaggeration of the patient's symptoms given as the reason for application for admittance to the mental hospital. The most frequent reasons for the urgent recommendation for admission to a mental institution were found to be: (1) lack of adequate training and understanding of the family physician who found himself unable to treat a disturbed and occasionally confused elderly patient; (2) lack of empathy and patience on the part of the family who considered, consciously or unconsciously, the geriatric patient as a burden and found it difficult to take time or make an effort to supervise him or give sufficient emotional support. Especially members of the younger generation, children and grandchildren, lacked understanding for the oldster's problems and eventually got vaguely apprehensive about things "going to happen to the grandchildren;" (3) denial of community support and neighborly help in some cases because it was thought to be too troublesome or not indicated; (4) the belief that the easiest way out of the situation was hospitalization of the patient in the nearest psychiatric institution where he would get adequate treatment or supervision; (5) the still common attitude among physicians and laymen in the United States that emotional disturbances are rarely curable and need to be treated in a closed psychiatric facility; and finally (6) the desperate economic condition of the elderly individual who may not have sufficient means to pay for a long period of psychiatric treatment. Often such people live alone, are left to their own devices, without anyone else's care, having to cook, shop and clean for themselves and tend feebly and apathetically to their own daily hygienic needs.

Many years of experience and study in psychiatric institutions have convinced me that many patients of the elderly age group were not originally in need of hospitalization and that others have been kept in such a hospital for many years after their remission from a psychotic episode. A great number of geriatric patients have received maximum hospital benefits and could be released from the phychiatric hospital. Others were actually returned to their families or put in foster or nursing homes to the surprise of other members of the patient's family or of the community who had "forgotten" the patient or lost interest, believing that rehabilitation in community or family life was not possible. Recently such a patient, even after 28 years of hospitalization, was released from hospitalization and adjusted himself well in the community. The release of this 64 year old former lawyer from hospitalization, being diagnosed as a "burned out schizophrenic" created great resistance on the part of the patient's brother and guardian, who did not "believe" in such an improvement in the patient and who was definitely afraid to be responsible for him.

It is quite possible that this situation might vary in different geographic areas and on different socioeconomic levels. A. Goldfarb (72) made an extensive study in several homes for the aged and in nursing homes in New York City and concluded that four out of five of all such aged persons, in the non-hospital institutions surveyed, were problems in management or were disturbing elements. At least one-third of them, according to psychiatric evaluation, would be eligible for admission to a state hospital by present standards, should a complaint or petition for such care be made. This demonstrates, according to Goldfarb, that the old age homes and nursing homes in the New York metropolitan area are acting as reservoirs of aged mentally disturbed persons and slow the flow of patients into mental hospitals. The state hospitals in New York State tend to receive persons who are qualitatively more anti-social and disruptive, or are confused, unmanageable and in need of terminal nursing and medical care.

There is no reason to doubt Goldfarb's findings and evaluations. It indicates only that the situation in New York City in regard to admission for hospitalization and psychiatric treatment in a psychiatric institution is different than in other states. First of all, it appears that the number of elderly persons with emotional disturbances is actually greater in relation to beds available in the state mental hospitals in New York City than in less urbanized areas. I also suspect that the economic conditions, including the housing conditions, in the greatest metropolitan area in the United States play a definite role in the placement and management of emotionally disturbed patients having problems of adjustment.

On the other hand, in the state of Kansas—which is primarily an agricultural state and where the housing problem is a minor factor and the economic condition seems to be more stabilized—other factors appear to be of greater importance.

A study of 105 geriatric patients, male and female, was undertaken at the Osawatomie State Hospital in Osawatomie, Kansas, on an outpatient basis. The study was started in September 1957 and ended August 1958. Of the 28 patients carefully examined during the first five-month period, only 7 were admitted to the hospital after careful examination at the Outpatient Department. These patients were either psychotic or suicidal or showed signs of a rather severe behavioral reaction and were found in need of hospitalization. Seven patients were sent to nursing homes for further care. The remaining 14 were returned to their families with special treatment recommendations to the family and the general practitioner who treated them before the referral to the hospital by court order for a 90-day observation period. They were admitted to the hospital but discharged the same day, after careful evaluation by the psychiatric social worker and a nurse. (154).

By August 1958, all 105 geriatric patients were evaluated on this outpatient basis. Of this number 50 were hospitalized (47%), 24 were sent to nursing homes (23%), and 31 were returned to their own family (30%). The patients sent to nursing homes belonged predominantly to the group of Chronic Brain Syndromes, associated with Cerebral Arteriosclerosis combined with physical handicaps in need of care and treatment which could not be given at home. Those who returned to their home environment were behavioral problems of a minor degree with occasional confusion, memory impairment, restlessness or reactive depression but without signs of a psychosis. They were treated by their family physician with tranquilizing medication or energizers under advice of the psychiatrist. In many cases of this kind, misunderstanding or wrong attitudes of other members of the family appeared to result in the precipitating stress producing these emotional disturbances.

A case history will best illustrate these observations and the correct procedure employed in this study:

The patient was a 75 year old, married, male janitor who was accompanied to the hospital by his wife and daughter. The social history revealed that the patient, during the past two years, frequently became angry and fought with his wife. He also wandered away from home and got lost. When found by the police, he could not understand why everyone was so excited and interested in his whereabouts. He had been treated by his family physician with tranquilizers. His wife was 51 years of age. This was the second marriage for both, having lasted 11 years to that time.

The patient came to our hospital because of a 90-day observation court order. At the interview he was friendly, cooperative, and answered questions willingly. He was neatly and cleanly dressed and was apparently used to taking good care of his personal appearance. His intellectual faculties were poor, however. He was not oriented to time or place and had a severe memory defect for recent and remote events. He believed himself to be 57 years old. He did not remember what he had eaten the day before. Although he had a fifth-grade education, he did not know how to multiply 9 times 9 and could not name the capital of his state. In his lifetime he never had a hobby of any kind except for participating in church activities. When asked to explain his wandering, he answered that he "just had to go" and did not know why. He liked to walk through the country, but he would always return. "I never want to go too far," he said. His thought processes were neither slow nor fast, and his thought content was not delusional. Hallucinations were not detected. Two months previous to the interview he started working as a janitor every night and seemed to like his job. He quit his job seven weeks later because of his confusion and wandering away and getting lost. He did not have insight into his condition and did not reveal any signs of anxiety. He denied worrying about money or anything else. When asked about his relationship with his wife, he answered, "I love my wife and I get along with her very fine."

Physical examination: Blood pressure was 180/90. There was a systolic murmur heard over the base of the heart that was not transmitted. The second aortic sound was accentuated and there were premature ventricular contractions. There was a cataract on the right eye and the left eye had had a cataract removed surgically. The neurological examination was normal. There were no other significant physical findings.

After the interview with the patient, the wife and the daughter, together with the social worker, were called into the office of the psychiatrist. The wife expressed disappointment in the marriage because she expected her husband to take care of her. This he had been able to do for the first few years until he grew older and less physically fit, so that he was gradually less able to continue satisfying her material needs. Bills for their new car and household items mounted until she had to go to work the preceding year in order to meet the expenses. Her work kept her away from home during the day, and his work kept him busy at night. These circumstances appeared to be the reason why the patient, who was left alone most of the day, became upset and wandered away from home. The psychiatrist explained that this situation had to be changed. The wife should stay at home more often than formerly and should give her husband more loving care in order to eliminate his feeling of loneliness and rejection. Otherwise the patient might become considerably more disturbed in the future. With these recommendations and the prescription of a tranquilizer for 10 days, the couple were sent home. A follow-up study of this patient after six months showed that he was well adjusted at home and not in need of further psychiatric help.

It has to be pointed out that follow-ups were necessary and had to be done on a monthly, three-month, or six-month basis. Four of the 105 geriatric patients belonging to an average age of 65 years continued to return once weekly to Outpatient treatment for group or individual psychotherapy regularly from three to six months. The patients transferred to nursing homes were carefully supervised by visits to the nursing homes by the social worker who was called when the patients got upset, disturbed, depressed, or showed any kind of management problem. Conferences between the nursing home administrators and the psychiatrist were frequent and eventually done through telephonic communication. Psychopharmacological drugs were given after contacting the general practitioner visiting the nursing homes. Occasionally a visit by the psychiatrist was found necessary for better observation of the patient in the nursing home or in the circle of his family and was done with the consent and common accord of the treating family physician. Such a communication system has been found of great importance and makes the treatment of the geriatric patient outside the hospital much easier. In addition, training courses in geriatric psychiatry were given at the hospital, under the supervision of the psychiatrist, with the help of all the members of the psychiatric team. These training courses, given about every four months at the hospital for about 10 nursing home administrators, helped definitely toward a better understanding of the geriatric patient's behavior and attitudes in the nursing home. Conferences and seminars were given on psychiatric problems of the elderly patient which soon awoke the interest of many general practitioners who came to observe and to learn.

It was remarkable that during the period from September 1957 to August 1958, 14 other applications for admission to this state mental institution were withdrawn by the family when appointments were given to evaluate the patient prior to admission. The reason for this withdrawal of the applications probably was the fact that hospitalization was not believed so urgently needed.

These are the observations of an eleven-month study at a Middle-West state institution in which overcrowding had been a tremendous problem previously. In this case we saw that the probate judges showed understanding and willingness to cooperate with the state institutions and the state government for a better treatment of the elderly citizen. I believe that the situation is similar in many other states and that careful pre-hospitalization evaluation of geriatric patients and treatment on an outpatient basis, combined with direct transfer of a certain number of patients to supervised and licensed nursing homes might be of definite value for the welfare of the elderly patient as well as for the community.

The results of my study therefore permit the following conclusions:

1. Definite admission procedures to psychiatric institutions should be deferred until after a 90-day observation and treatment period.
2. Evaluation by a psychiatric team prior to admission of the geriatric patient is necessary and of value.
3. Treatment on an outpatient basis for geriatric patients with emotional problems should be given when indicated.
4. Better rapport between the hospital psychiatrist and the family physician referring the patient for hospitalization is needed.
5. Nursing home administrators should receive training at the psychiatric hospital in order to be able to understand and handle more efficiently the problems of the aged.
6. The services of all community resources such as Senior Citizens Clubs, Day Centers and Volunteer organizations should be optimally utilized.
7. The psychiatric team should gain a good picture of the economic condition as well as the emotional background of the family environment of the patient prior to the requested hospitalization.
8. Rapport and frequent communications between the hospitals' psychiatric team and the staffs of the nursing or old age homes are vital.

5

THE TREATMENT IN A PSYCHIATRIC HOSPITAL

A. INDIVIDUAL PSYCHOTHERAPY

It is well known that S. Freud (60) did not favor individual psychotherapy for patients over 45 years of age. He believed that after that age the patient's character would not be flexible enough to make the necessary personality changes demanded of him once he has gained insight into his condition. Memory disturbances also were believed to represent an obstacle to treatment because the elderly patients might not be able to recall details of their childhood which would be important for the analysis. Fenichel (54) and other outstanding psychotherapists therefore preferred not to treat geriatric patients with individual psychotherapy and became, to a certain degree, responsible for the pessimistic attitude taken by psychoanalysts that geriatric patients can hardly be helped by individual psychotherapy.

K. Abraham (1), however, in 1919 became skeptical of this hopeless attitude of the psychoanalysts and believed that the age of the neurosis was more important than the age of the patient. He successfully analyzed four neurotic patients about 50 years of age.

S. E. Jelliffee (84) also published satisfactory results with psychoanalytic treatment of elderly patients and concluded that chronological, physiological and psychological age do not go hand in hand. F. Alexander (4), modifying psychoanalytic technique and emphasizing two different forms of individual psychotherapy, insight therapy and supportive therapy, recommends treatment of elderly patients with individual psychotherapy where the Egostrength is sufficient to handle insight-directed interpretations. He has successfully used individual psychotherapy with older patients.

Kaufman (90) believes that the emotional rigidity found in so many elderly persons is more a defense mechanism than an irreversible condition and is therefore amenable to treatment. He has successfully treated two geriatric patients suffering from psychotic depressions. He warns, however, not to generalize his findings and agrees partially with Fenichel that, in cases of physically disabled patients, the neurosis might be the best form of adjustment and therefore psychotherapy would be unsuccessful unless some external changes of the life situation would be possible. The importance of the possibility of changing certain life situations was also emphasized by Alexander and French (4) who found problems in connection with retirement, for instance, a great handicap in helping their elderly patients with individual psychotherapy.

M. Grotjahn (74) has also successfully treated emotionally disturbed geriatric patients with individual psychotherapy. He thinks that resistance against unpleasant insight is lessened in old age and that even "narcissistic threats" for the Ego become acceptable. Grotjahn assumes that depression and guilt in the older patient can be relieved with the same techniques as in younger patients through the correction of misconceptions and unrealistic anticipation, as, for instance, the belief that old people are beyond sin and sex. The elderly subject must go through a reverse Oedipus situation where not the son fears the father but the aging father the son. He must work through his unconscious relation to his son. Psychoanalytic therapy has been shown, according to Grotjahn, to be effective by interpretation of this situation and by helping the patient gain insight.

Meerloo (113), by analytically oriented psychotherapy, was able to help elderly patients rediscover hidden inner resources and thus to conquer their feelings of uselessness and boredom. He describes how a 76 year old former lawyer with great memory defects started, during therapy, to study philosophy as a new hobby. With this new-found detachment from subjective complaints, he obtained a clearer grasp of the subject of logic than previously. Meerloo emphasizes the importance of environmental factors in the aged and also recommended treatment of the marriage partner or of the children when necessary. He does not recommend analysis of the resistance of the patient, since such an analysis might stir up psychotic features. He believes that the therapist as a transference figure has to replace a real loss of love and social appreciation. Carefully chosen interpretation, according to Meerloo, has, however, the same clarifying value as in the treatment of psychoneurosis in younger persons.

J. Weinberg (149) modifies traditional and analytic techniques and uses a more active and less formalistic approach to individual psychotherapy with the aged. He maintains that the therapist has to enter more freely into a relationship with the patient and also to manipulate, if necessary, the environment in which the older person lives. This may range from educating the family, friends, and those who are entrusted with the care of the aged concerning their needs and the detection of symptoms, to a dogged gnawing at the conscience of society to provide the necessities for a better emotional climate for our aging population.

G. J. Wayne (147) reaffirms this more active approach in geriatric psychotherapy and favors not only directing the course of therapy but also providing reassuring discussion, guidance and even environmental manipulation where indicated. He also feels that certain educational techniques, such as realistic discussions of the cultural attitude toward the aged, can be useful.

A. J. Goldfarb (70, 71) has used a very different technique of individual psychotherapy with geriatric patients and has reported good results. His patients were treated with brief and widely spaced sessions. The maximum length of sessions was 15 minutes. The aim in each session was to provide emotional gratification of the patient and to increase his self-esteem. The therapist took the role of the protective parent who was strong and powerful and able to help the patient. Goldfarb recommends seeing geriatric patients twice within the first week and afterwards as infrequently as possible. The patients are being "fed" emotionally and obtain strength from the therapist. After each session they tend to feel stronger. In this way the patients win over the potentially threatening authority figure as an ally. When he verbalizes his resentment against the therapist but is able to win the therapist's protection all the same by "defeating him," the geriatric patient feels more powerful and to be gaining strength. Goldfarb considers it important to explain the patient's difficulties to his medical, administrative and social service staff by means of staff conferences and uses the staff's assistance to reinforce the results of his individual psychotherapy. According to Goldfarb, this method was not effective in psychotic patients but was of value for psychoneurotic disorders of the aged and for patients suffering from acute and even chronic brain syndromes. In this way, many of his patients could be treated in a home for the aged and infirm and did not need to be transferred to a psychiatric institution.

Since 1954, I have been able to treat a number of geriatric patients of both sexes in psychiatric institutions. I used the "Brief Therapy" recommended by Goldfarb on psychiatric wards and found it effective and useful with elderly patients suffering from acute and chronic brain syndromes associated with cerebral arteriosclerosis, with senility, chronic alcoholism, central nervous system syphilis (after the end of their specific antiluetic treatment) and with geriatric patients suffering from neurological disorders of various kinds. This technique definitely helped these patients to gain Egostrength by increasing their self-esteem, by verbalizing their resentment and anger. Most notably helped were patients who were management problems on the ward by being upset, excited, threatening to other patients and to personnel; patients with poor toilet and eating habits; and others suffering from depressive features and refusing to eat. This form of treatment also brought a few delusional patients nearer reality. It was also of use in encouraging listless and apathetic patients to participate with greater interest in recreational and occupational activities and to further their socializaion and rehabiliation program.

This form of therapy tended to decrease the dosage of tranquilizing medication given to patients to improve their adjustment on the ward. Occasionally, delusional patients could be induced finally to participate in group psychotherapy sessions.

It was found difficult, however, to make an exact controlled study of the value of this form of individual psychotherapy on a psychiatric ward. Members of my staff reported relapses of emotional disturbances of my patients after visits of relatives, after receiving mail or after physical sickness, so frequent in the elderly population. For this reason, it was found difficult frequently to state exactly to what degree "Brief Psychotherapy" was the real cause of the improvement or what other factors were involved.

Individual psychoanalytic oriented psychotherapy was given by myself to 14 patients in a psychiatric hospital with relatively favorable results. Six of these were treated on an outpatient basis at the Galesburg State Research Hospital (Illinois) for an average period of four months. Eight were treated at Osawatomie State Hospital (Kansas). Three of these eight patients had been hospitalized for behavioral problems. The other five received treatment on an outpatient basis at the Geriatric Treatment and Research Unit at Osawatomie State Hospital for five to seven months. The average age of the patients was 65 years. Of these 14 patients, 10 were males; 4 were females. All of them were treated in individual sessions of 50 minutes' duration, once a week. The diagnoses included Chronic Brain Syndrome, associated with Cerebral Arteriosclerosis, with features of depression: 2; Chronic Brain Syndrome, associated with Cerebral Arteriosclerosis, with behavioral reaction: 2; Chronic Brain Syndrome, associated with Senility, with behavioral reaction: 2; Chronic Brain Syndrome, associated with Alcoholism, with neurotic reaction: 2; Psychoneurosis, severe, anxiety reaction: 3; Psychoneurosis, depressive reaction, moderately severe: 3.

From this group of 14 patients treated by psychoanalytic oriented individual psychotherapy, 8 improved remarkably and 2 slightly, while 4 patients discontinued the individual sessions after six months of treatment without positive results. The hospitalized patients continued with their previous activities but no new occupational or recreational therapy was added for them in order to facilitate control.

A case history of a patient of mine on the Geriatric Unit at Osawatomie State Hospital (Kansas) in 1955, treated by 14 sessions of individual psychotherapy well illustrates my method, its difficulties and problems, and final results.

CASE HISTORY

This is the case history of a 62 year old, widowed, female patient suffering from Psychoneurosis, Anxiety Reaction, severe, for which she was hospitalized on voluntary basis in a state mental hospital in Kansas. The diagnosis was made by psychiatric examination and psychological testing. It was decided to treat the patient by individual psychotherapy only. Tranquilizing drugs or any other medication was not given. The individual psychotherapy was done by myself for the duration of 50 minutes, once a week. After each session, a report was made. The patient improved considerably after 14 sessions of individual psychotherapy. She was much quieter, able to sleep well, felt hopeful, more secure of herself, and left the hospital to take care of the household for one of her brothers and her brother's grandson. She was told to return to the hospital if and when her symptoms bothered her again. She was urged to write monthly reports about her adjustments and her feelings. After four months, a letter was received in which she let me know that she felt fine, that she had no difficulties in adjusting to her new situation, that she slept well and was praised by her brother for taking such good care of the household. Afterwards, nothing was heard from her. About one year later, news was received at the hospital by one of her neighbors who was hospitalized that the patient continued to do well.

Individual Psychotherapy Session 1

In the patient's first session she was eager to talk, was very restless and revealed remarkable trembling of her hands. She complained of being nervous and of being unable to sleep at night. She could join in activities but was upset easily and talked about another patient having a crying spell the day before, which upset and frightened her. Furthermore, she complained about being unable to concentrate. She worried about her hair not being combed, about the heat, and said, "I have a pounding in the insides." She kept her experiences "bottled up." She talked about the treatment she had at another hospital where she had 11 electric shock treatments. She was frightened of this. She was "dismissed unimproved." "They could not do anything for me." She said that she was especially afraid of electric shock treatment because she noticed that blood vessels on the thigh of another patient had burst during treatment. She remarked that she felt more confused and nervous in the morning. In the middle of the session, she started to talk about her father who had died six years previously. When her father died, she stayed with her brother and also took care of two little boys, aged four and eight, who were children of neighbors. When the family of the boys moved out of town, she got arthritis. She consulted a psychiatrist who advised her to develop a hobby or other interest. However, she felt unable to do so. She talked about another patient on the ward who helped her to make her bed and upon whom she was very dependent. She expressed ambivalence about her being at a state hospital. She had dreaded coming there. "My folks," she said, "wanted me to go to a nursing home." She complained about her lack of sleep and asked the therapist if she was "hopeless." At the end of the interview she agreed to come weekly to the therapist's office "because I like to help me and to help you." She felt she got worse all the time. She could not take a bath by herself and had to be helped by the nurse.

Comment:

This patient suffered from a lifelong anxiety reaction which became worse after the death of her father. Besides her anxiety and extreme restlessness, it was felt that her hostility was hidden but great. She was a very dependent, passive person who needed the help of others and the support of the hospital for her own feelings of inadequacy. After the death of her father, she seemed to have lost all goal in life.

Individual Psychotherapy Session 2

The patient showed less anxiety and less restlessness during the second session. She continued to talk freely about her problems but tried to be evasive when her relationship to her father and mother was mentioned.

She started to talk about the movie on the ward which disturbed her because she did not like to see men fighting. She did not dare to leave because "I am afraid to get the worst of it." She talked about her two brothers and said that she took care of their children; but it did not seem that her "brothers had an important part in her life." She mentioned that she took care of her father after the death of her mother. Her father lived to be 91 years old. She repeated twice that "he had a wonderful disposition and I am a little bit like him." Her mother had died 15 years before, because of heart trouble, and, even before her mother's death, she took care of her father who could not dress himself and was weak. She bathed him frequently because he liked to be bathed by her, and he often refused to be washed by his wife with whom he quarreled frequently. "My father looked nice when he was clean. He looked better than most other men." After the death of her father, she had a nervous breakdown because she did not know what to live for. She said that she had many misunderstandings with her mother, but she did not give further information.

She also talked about her marriage and her divorce. Her husband was a salesman in a factory where she had worked as a secretary. She knew him for four years before marriage but denied having a sexual relationship before marriage. She felt bad about the divorce because she was a Lutheran and did not believe in divorce. She never tried to marry again.

She had economic worries during her marriage because her husband lost everything on the stock market during the depression in 1929. He then went to live with his mother, but she did not find this agreeable. She never had children. She did not want to have children and neither did her husband. "I never felt able to take the responsibilities." Her husband used preventative methods to keep from having children.

She remarked that she developed arthritis during the last two years when she took care of her father. After his death, she went to a medical center to get treatment for her arthritis but had to discontinue the treatment because the medicine was "too expensive."

At the end of the interview she said that she worried too much, that she could not smile, and that she was ashamed of being in a mental institution. "I feel I cannot face people when I am in a place like this. I can't relax."

Remarks:

It became more evident that this patient was a passive, immature person who never was able to take responsibilities and did not dare to have children. The symptoms of her arthritis started when she took care of her father. In spite of her assurances that she loved him very deeply, it was felt that she started to feel overworked and overburdened at that time but did not dare to express her hostile feelings against the father, to whom she had a life-long emotional and erotic attachment.

Individual Psychotherapy Session 3

The patient came to my office trembling and very anxious. Both of her hands shook, but she immediately began to talk. She wanted some medicine to help her overcome her shaking and stated that she was much afraid of getting electric shock treatment. She said that electric shock treatment helped her at a medical center at the beginning, but then the doctors said that it would not help her further. She mentioned that she got upset on the previous day when one patient hit another patient with a drinking cup. The dayroom was so crowded that it was hard for her to sit there. If the other ladies went to bed, they went to sleep immediately, but she could not. She was afraid of not getting well and of staying at the hospital for a long time. She was afraid because that day was "Friday the thirteenth." Some people were superstitious because it brought bad luck to them.

Then she talked about her husband. He had died last summer, but it did not even "bother her a little bit." Her marriage was something unpleasant; she would have liked to forget it. Her husband got "awfully cross" when he lost on the stock market. "He fussed at me quite a lot." Before marriage he was good, also to her folks, but afterwards he thought she did not love him anymore. "We had to stay with his mother; she was old and cranky." "I told him we should have a place of our own." But her mother-in-law needed attention. For one year the patient cooked all the mother-in-law's meals. The mother-in-law did not want the husband to "give me any attention and did not like him putting his arms around me." She felt sorry for her mother-in-law because she was old and childish. She never spoke a cross word to her.

"I feel my marriage was a mistake. If I had kept on working I might not have had this nervous breakdown." Her husband was generous with his money. They were married for 11 years; she married at 32 and was divorced at 43. Then she had forgotten her shorthand. "I was afraid to apply for another position." She stayed with her father and mother. She mentioned that she had many dates before marriage but never had she really been in love. Her husband was a nice looking and very popular man. He belonged to a club and left her alone many nights. "I waited a long time in my car for him, watching the people go by." Now she could not sit that long any more. Her husband, she said, was always in the company of men and frequently picked her up after a movie. She believed, however, her marriage was a happy one; and as a Lutheran, she did not believe in divorce. She did confess, however, that she did not go to church enough. "I feel badly about it now. I feel that I am getting punished for it. If I would have been a good Christian, it would not have happened."

Then she talked again about being afraid of electric shock treatment. She remarked that she was also afraid of doctors although she realized that doctors tried to help. "I am afraid to spend the rest of my life at the hospital. I want to leave here, but I want to get well before that."

At the end of the interview she inquired of the therapist what she had to do during the day.

Comments:

On different occasions the patient mentioned being afraid of men and women alike. She apparently did not like to take care of her mother-in-law but never could express hostility. She remarked that her marriage was unhappy but she still could not express her resentment toward her husband who apparently was more interested in male company. Finally she again showed her dependent attitude by wanting the therapist to tell her what to do and what not to do during the day.

Individual Psychotherapy Session 4

The patient was less upset and restless when she entered the office and showed less tremor of her hands. She started to talk about doctors. She was afraid of them because she might get hurt, but then she corrected herself and remarked, "I know quite well that doctors only try to help." Walking was more difficult for her than before and she hoped that the massage she had gotten might help her. She asked for permission to drink a coke in the therapist's office, and while she did she appeared to be more relaxed than she had been the previous time. Then she said that she had no patience to sit through a movie. She also had a horror of being "locked up or tied in a chair." She was unable to smile, she remarked, because she had nothing to live for or to smile at. She also did not want people to know that she was in an "Insane Asylum." "It is a disgrace." She was wondering if the people who were hospitalized had ever been bright before. She had worked as a secretary for the assistant manager and had liked her work. She made mistakes but was never criticized for them. She was wondering how long she had to stay here. She pointed out that she had been disappointed when she had first come here. She could not stand the "elderly ladies," and she felt sorry that one of the patients had left for home.

Then she talked about her mother. She had died 15 years ago and was very strict. Once when she was 16, she wanted to go to a party, but her mother would not let her. When she wanted to ask Dad about it, her mother said that Dad had nothing to do with it. Both of her parents were born in the "old country" and people over there were very moralistic. She spent two years with an uncle who was a minister. He, too, had not been born in the United States and was minister to a church for 25 years. Her mother never talked about sex; it was forbidden at home. But when she was 17, she read a book about it. She never knew a man before her marriage. Her husband had to support her and she had to stay at home. "Times have changed now."

Her father liked people. "I have a good disposition just like my father. He passed away in 1951. I took care of him and even shaved him." She always kept house for him. He got up at 5 a.m. She prepared his pipe and his breakfast. Her husband was a wonderful man, too. He took care of all the bills. She never had to make decisions. "I feel that I am nervous because I cannot depend on anyone now." Her two brothers, she said, also helped her continuously. Now she could not even make her own bed. She had "arthritis" and could not move. She could not do any cooking. Her sickness came when her father passed away. Her brothers spoiled her. She hated to get up at 6 a.m. here. She did not know what to do all day long. "I am afraid of going to pieces. I sometimes feel that if I could scream it would be better. But I am afraid they will take me to one of the seclusion rooms." She had to walk up and down. She could not eat in the dining room. She could not stay long enough with other people.

At the end of the session she smiled at the therapist, said that he was a "nice man," and asked him how long he had been in the United States and where he came from.

Comment:

The first sign of a positive transference became evident. The patient was less restless, talked freely about her problems, and began to get some insight into her condition. She realized that her dependency upon others had something to do with her nervousness. She tried to identify with her father whom she bathed and shaved. Did she want him to be a woman? Her Superego was strong and she controlled her hostility. Her "arthritis" was to be considered a defense mechanism. (There was no clinical evidence for rheumatoid arthritis.)

Individual Psychotherapy Session 5

When the patient entered the therapist's office, she was more tense and anxious than she had been the last time. She started to talk about the walk she had taken the previous day with the group. She noted that she could neither sit or stand still, but that it was nice and shady outside. She said she was scared every time she had to see a "doctor." She was afraid of getting hurt. She hoped to get medicine. She could not sleep without medicine. It bothered her to eat in the dining room. She could have better table manners. She said that she still enjoyed a good movie but that she did not care for "Wild West" pictures.

"I feel so helpless; I feel somebody has to be with me all the time to help me. I feel in the morning I need somebody to comb my hair. I always worry so much."

Then she spoke about the time she attended school and also when she moved to a farm. After finishing school, she stayed two years at home and took care of her mother. Her teachers, she said, were very nice and one of them was Swedish. She believed that she was unable to smile. When she heard the nurses laughing and saw them smiling, she wished that she could have their health. "If I could laugh and forget myself, I would be fine." She was "better off" than the other patients on the ward who had to be waited on hand and foot. Then she said she might not be able to leave the hospital. She worried that she might not be able to see her folks next Sunday. She remarked that another patient seemed not to be getting better. "When she cannot be helped, I cannot be helped, either." She was frightened of everything, especially of male patients. They cursed so much. Her toe hurt her so much that she could hardly walk. Her lower plate caused her to have a sore mouth. She wanted to get well, however. She liked it better in this building than when she first came to the hospital. She helped in the dining room but could not move fast enough. Then she talked about her mother. Her mother had "a severe look." She felt that she looked more like the mother now. She considered that she had been a burden to her brother and did not want to become one again. "Some people, when they get mad, they curse. I am a Christian; I cannot do it. I am all bottled up inside. I feel I could scream, but I take my suffering in silence." She did not keep things clean enough. Her mother and brother reproved her for this. She felt agitated. She would like to get away soon, but she could not take care of herself.

At the end of the interview she repeated that she would not be able to talk to her folks next Sunday.

Comment:

The patient was more nervous than she had been at the previous session. Her ambivalence became evident in regard to staying in or leaving the hospital. She had more somatic complaints than before. The visit of her relatives on the next Sunday had a remarkable influence on this session.

Individual Psychotherapy Session 6

The patient came into the office more relaxed than the last time. She complained about having a sore throat and said she felt "impatient." She had waited for her folks, but they had not come the day before although she had on her best dress and had done her hair well. She remarked that the preceding Decoration Day she had driven to the cemetery. There she had decorated her father's and her mother's graves. This time she was not able to go. She felt too nervous. She hated to lose her father. He was feeble and got up many times at night. Sometimes she herself had to get up every hour. But she liked to do this. Everybody liked her father and he had a large funeral. "It made me happy that he had so many friends."

Then she talked about her mother. At her funeral there were not too many people present. Her mother suffered from varicose veins, but her death came as a blow. Her mother, she said, was cranky with her. She did not want her to go with boys. Instead, she had to go to Sunday school. Her younger brother did not approve of her smoking. He believed that she did not keep the house clean enough. Her mother did not approve of parties at night. When they had parties in her own home, the mother always had to see what was going on. Her mother wanted her "to be associated only with high-class people." She was a strict mother. She had her first date when she was 17. "My mother did not trust me. Sometimes my father said I could go, but my mother did not want it." Father and Mother, she said, frequently quarreled about it. Her mother was cranky with Dad, too. She always wanted him to change clothes when he went to town. However, he complied only when the patient intervened. She did not hate her mother. Nonetheless, she felt that mothers should be more lenient. Her father drank whisky occasionally. Her mother did not approve of drinking.

She never kissed boys before she was 23 years old, and then

only goodnight, after a movie. People went in streetcars at this time and not by automobiles. She was afraid to kiss a boy because it might lead to something else. "I never was very affectionate." She felt that she was pretty as a girl. She described herself as having light brown hair and always being neatly dressed. But she did not want to get married. She liked her job too much. Every vacation and holiday she went home to help her mother. "I never kissed my father." Her father did not like to kiss her, either. She had several proposals before she was 32, but she did not want to marry a farmer. "I was a highbrow," she said, "and my chances were better in a big city." She really loved her husband. At 32 people called her "a mere angel child." She looked younger than her age. She liked to earn money and to be independent. This, she said, was the reason that she did not want to marry earlier.

She was afraid of becoming a cripple because of her arthritis. Rheumatic arthritis could not be cured, she said. She got injections for it in the past, but they did not help. "I put up a good front. I feel that I could go to pieces. I am hiding my feelings from you. I am afraid that I will get electric shock treatment. I got them at the medical center. I feel that I am punished now and will never get into Heaven."

Comment:

The patient was less tense and anxious. On the ward she related herself better to other female patients and was more interested in occupational therapy. In this session she expressed hostility against her strict mother. She revealed herself as an inhibited person who, even at the age of 32, suffered from an Oedipus complex. She rationalized liking her job better than getting married. She revealed a great attachment to her father. Father and daughter avoided kissing each other. Her severe Superego helped her to control herself. It is to be hoped that the true reasons for her failure in marriage will become more evident.

Individual Psychotherapy Session 7

The patient entered the office somewhat trembling and depressed and starting talking about a cold. She had received aspirin and nose drops for it. She had to perspire so much. She remarked that she was "frightened to come to the interview today." "If I do not give a correct answer, something drastic has to happen." Electric shock treatment might have to be started, she felt.

Her brother had been here today, she remarked. She was happy to see her brother and cried when he left. This was the first time she had cried since her father's death. She had a feeling of being unable to leave this institution, but she tried to be optimistic about it. She read in the newspaper that the methods of treatment in Kansas were excellent. She told her brother that she was feeling better but that she still felt nervous. She took a ride with him in his car. When she returned she felt "kind of blue." The ladies in the wheel chair and the other ones, old ones, were pitiful to look at. She did not see that there was any hope for them as there was hope for her. "I would like to be free from these nerves, but I do not have the willpower to do things." She had been here for three months now, she said. She could not keep up with the exact date but many other patients could not do so, either. At night she had a pain across her chest. First she thought it was her heart. She was taught, however, that this pain was simply caused by nerves. The morning nurse was really sympathetic with her; she had known her for a long time.

Then she talked about her uncle (her mother's brother) who had given her a good education and had sent her to high school. She had to quit, however, because she had to go home to help her mother. She did not realize at that time that an education was more important than helping her mother. She was only 13. Her uncle did not take sides and left it up to her to go home or not. She took care of her father also. "You get used to hanging, too, they say."

She always had it easy and never had to go through what she was going through now. She believed that she should not be such a baby. Then she remarked that she looked like a tramp, but she would like to have her hair fixed. She was told that she was very attractive and she always had nice clothes. Once she had plenty of money, but now she had none.

Comment:

The visit of her brother did not disturb her much, but by her somatic complaints she let the therapist know that she was unable to leave the hospital yet. She felt more secure in the hospital environment and started to gain some insight. She realized that she was immature and liked to get attention by her good looks. By taking better care of her personal appearance, she began to show some improvement. Remarking that she "got used to taking care of her father," she also began to express some of her repressed hostility. She might, however, have shifted the responsibility of taking care of her from her brother to the hospital. It remains to be seen if her brother's visit will not awaken deeper feelings in her at some future time.

Individual Psychotherapy Session 8

The patient entered the office trembling, but after a while she became quiet. "It pounds inside and outside," she said. She did not know why she trembled so much. The nurses turned the light on at night, and she couldn't sleep. When she was awake, it took her several hours to sleep again. She thought at night how long she would have to stay here and what kind of treatment she would get. Some patients told her that it was difficult to get out of here. Maybe medicine would help her. She was afraid all the time but did not know what the reason for this fear was. She was afraid of the doctors. Doctors punish people, unknowingly. She had punishment coming to her. She always had been nervous. She was nervous even before her marriage. Marriage was a serious step and a crucial one in her life. She did not believe in divorce. When she looked for a job, she was always nervous, even though she only went by recommendation. She did not like dictation at night. She was afraid that she could not read it the next day. Her husband was older than she, and she had always been dependent on him. He became irritable and angry when he lost all his money.

She was also afraid of lightning, car accidents and of any changes in her address. The arthritis caused her breakdown. She hated to be crippled. Now she could not wear beautiful shoes as she always liked to do. If she had no arthritis, she could dress better. She was not able to fight her arthritis. She gave up. She was also frightened of talking to people. She was afraid of "not making good." Once she was married, she could not go back to her old position. She did not fight with people. Her brother told her that she could not fool a doctor. When her parents died, she could depend on her brother. She was worried about the interview, too. The therapist might lock her up. She never could hurt herself or others. She believed people always "walked over her." She did not mean anyone in particular. If she finally left the hospital, she would try to stay on her own feet. Here at the hospital they helped her. Her brother said she was too spoiled. She was worried about tomorrow. She felt bitter about being at the hospital. It was a punishment. She should fight more to get out. She was afraid to eat with other people. She could not write to any one of her relatives. She was afraid she might spend all the rest of her life at the hospital.

Comment:

Again, there were some signs of insight, but her anxiety remained great and the emotional display was partially of hysterical nature. Her "arthritis" served two purposes for her: (1) to have a reason to be taken care of and (2) to avoid expression of her hostility which was great. The therapeutic progress is slow.

Individual Psychotherapy Session 9

The patient showed resistance at coming to the interview. "I have told you everything and do not know what more to talk about." It frightened her to talk to many people. She was scared of the staff meeting she would have next Wednesday. Everything was confused; she was worried about what would become of her. She did not think she had a bright future. She would like to have her mother and her father back. She regretted what she had done to them. She should have been more thoughtful. Her mother, for instance, did not want her to smoke cigarettes or to play cards. Her arthritis and her worries caused her nervous breakdown. She did not want to go to a nursing home, either. There she would not be able to have a doctor when she needed one. She did not think that she was improving. She could not marry, either, because she was not attractive any more. The days were so long. She dreaded the hot weather. She felt "like a prisoner condemned to die." She kept in contact with two friends of hers with whom she worked when she was a secretary. She wished that the therapist could cure her nerves and that she could go home. She would like to be a companion to an elderly lady, but now she could not even take care of herself. She did not look nice any more and could not walk because of her arthritis. She was afraid to come to the interview. When she was asked if she would like to continue talking to the therapist or if she would rather have the interviews discontinued, she said she would like to continue talking about her troubles.

Comment:

The patient's ambivalence became more evident. She felt threatened to leave. However, she was less upset and restless than before and on the ward began taking part, although with ambivalence, in ward activities. This ambivalence was interpreted to her, and she agreed with the interpretation.

Individual Psychotherapy Session 10

The patient entered the office agitated. She had visitors the day before. Her younger brother, his wife, her niece and nephew came to see her. She looked forward to seeing them, and when they left she cried a little. But at times she feared seeing them again. Last night she had slept well for the first time. However, the therapist did not realize what bad shape she was in, she remarked. She could scream but she did not dare. She would like to be a companion to an old lady. It frightened her to come to the therapist's office. She was hurt once by a dentist. Patients told her once they got in here they did not leave anymore, but Mrs. .... and Mrs. .... left all the same. They were less nervous than she was, however. Maybe she did not have enough faith. Her brother told her she should not think continuously of her troubles. She would like to "blow her top." She was afraid of "getting wild." She could not lie down and relax as other patients did. If she would not wake up in the morning any more, she would be happy. Her brother's children interested her, especially her brother's grandchild. When she first suffered from arthritis, she gave up, quit working in the household. That was wrong. She could not cry and she could not smile. She wondered why the therapist was able to smile. The attendants told her she was fussing too much. She got more attention than most of the others, they told her. She worried again about Sunday when her relatives would come. When she was well, she had her hair nicely fixed and wore a beautiful dress. She did not like the day hall and the "old men" in there.

Comment:

In this interview the patient was full of contradictions; however, she revealed interest in her brother's children and in her brother's grandchild. When her brother came to visit her, she received him in a beautiful new dress. She smiled at seeing her brother's grandchild and greeted it with joy. She slept well, looked more relaxed, started to eat more and gained weight.

Individual Psychotherapy Session 11

The patient entered the office in an anxious state. She said, "I believe it is a long, drawn-out affair." She felt impatient because she was at the hospital three months now and she could not get over her nervousness. She could not keep up with her looks and with her dress. She got many kinds of food she did not like, but she liked to drink milk. Changes would upset her. It made her sad to see her younger brother and his wife. They came to visit her. The other patients were not clean and cursed a lot in the day hall. Her arthritis did not permit her to walk. She could not wear shoes. She took people's troubles too much to heart. She made friends with another patient on arrival. She got along fine with her. Mrs. .... cursed a lot when she did not help her in the dining room and worked too slow. She was even too slow walking on the grounds. If her brother would come today, she would not be ready to leave. Nerves are hard to cope with. The afternoon attendants were pretty tough. She was scared for the next day to come. She knew a lot of important people once. She had many good friends, but after her divorce she resented men generally. She did not trust men any more. She did not get such a good deal as she expected. Her father and her mother were hurt when they knew about it. She liked a man to be neat, good-looking and well educated. Maybe her ideas were too high. She could not face people after having been in a mental institution. She had to get over her nervous condition. Worry about her arthritis brought it on. At her birthday party, "elderly ladies" started to dance. It was disgusting to her. She was worried about how her hair was going to look. The afternoon nurses seemed to be cranky with her. She was worried about her table manners. She did not lose contact. She believed the therapist might be able to understand her and to help her more. She shook so much. Maybe God punished her for not being a good Christian.

Comment:

Patient started to verbalize more hostility. She began to get more interested in her personal appearance, made friends more easily. Her thoughts began to concentrate on her brother, his family, her brother's grandchild, on a life outside the hospital. Her anxiety is decreasing. Signs of a positive transference are evident.

Individual Psychotherapy Session 12

The patient entered the office of the therapist more composed and less restless than on former occasions. She complained about being unable to sleep and not having an appetite. She worried about having lost a dress in the laundry and now she preferred to wash her dresses herself. She was, however, unable to iron them by herself. Other patients asked to go home, but she felt that she wasn't ready yet. Everything started with her arthritis. Her brother had no room for her. She always felt she had to lean on somebody. She could not be of any help now. She worried about her hair and her looks. She could not be happy. She had a number of disappointments. She would have been better off if she had continued with her office work. It was a mistake to get married. She was in love with her husband. Many boys wanted to marry her, but they were farmers only and she did not like to live on a farm. Her mother trembled and so did her younger brother. Her shaking was a family affair. Her father was very calm. The occupational therapist wanted her to do some painting. She was not good at that. She cared for reading only. She was especially interested in politics and read all the political articles in the newspaper. She had nothing to live for.

The last work she did was to take care of a little boy. His parents were dancers and now they were working for a Murray studio. She took the little boy to church. She felt unable to work now. She could not cook any more. She could not even prepare breakfast. She used to bake bread and a good pie, but she forgot how to do everything. She was too dependent. She could not get interested in anything. Other patients were looking nicer than she was.

Comment:

The patient started on an occupational therapy project, then discontinued, but was able to do some painting a few days later. She now dresses nicely. She started to get interested in cooking and baking and talked to the kitchen helpers. Her interest in taking care of her brother's grandchild becomes a realistic possibility. She sleeps well at night. The therapist encouraged her to take part in new occupational activities, praised her and complimented her on her good looks. She indeed looked 10 years younger than on arrival at the hospital 3½ months ago. She also started to become more interested in local and world politics.

Individual Psychotherapy Session 13

The patient entered the office complaining about the heat. She always had to carry something like a fan with her. She lost her appetite. She felt that she had not improved. She could not relax. It was difficult for her to come to the hall and do some sewing and painting. There was so much commotion. The "elderly ladies" at the dance were out of their senses. They seemed to be happy and not nervous. She wondered how long she had to stay. She could not understand why other people went home. Three ladies from her room left already. She remembered things better than they did. But the others did not get excited so much. She could now go to the dining room to eat without being scared. She was scared of doctors and "higher up people" only. She was afraid to get lost in the city where her brother lived. It was a disgrace to come to a "place like this." A "real high-class person" did not lose her mind. She never had any desire to hit anyone, but she could not sit still. She was more of a problem than anybody else. There was nothing wrong with her physically. It was "just nerves." The nurses seemed to be happy, but she felt bitter. She was scared to see her brother again. She could not make a good appearance. She was proud and she wanted to look nice. Talking with the therapist helped her. She could let the therapist know how sick she was. Her nervous breakdown came from worry. She had arthritis. She was afraid of becoming a cripple. She could not do any sewing, either. It was not that she did not want to, but she could not.

Comment:

The patient continues to show improvement. She started to sew in the day hall and read newspapers daily. She got interested in painting but still needed encouragement. Her "arthritis" got better without medication. She was able to move the fingers of both hands.

Individual Psychotherapy Session 14

The patient entered the office in a natural way and offered the therapist a coke to drink, complaining about the hot weather. She said that she expected her brother to come to the hospital next Sunday to take her with him. She remarked that she did not like her brother but she was interested in his grandchild, a boy now five years old who would be in need of a "better education" than her brother and his wife could offer him. She was not needed here, anyway, and did not like to stay in a room with other "old ladies" any more. Her friends at the hospital had already left, and she did not have any news from them. She did not like to be forgotten. Her arthritis got better anyway, perhaps the heat helped her hands. She perspired such a lot. The attendants told her off. They seemed to believe that she was able to do a lot of things but did not want to. She did not like to dance with the "old men" because they would ruin her new dress. The therapist alone understood her. She knew now that she did not like her mother too well and wanted to take care of her Dad alone but mother did not let her. Her husband was nice, but he was never so intelligent as father was. Maybe she could still find another husband. She did not feel too old yet. Everybody told her how young she looked. And she was a good cook once and would like to try cooking again.

Remarks:

On the Sunday following this therapy session, the patient's brother came and took her home for a trial visit to take care of his household and his grandchild who lived in an apartment nearby together with his parents. The therapist gave permission for the trial visit by phone and did not talk to the patient. The patient was discharged from trial visit after a waiting period of nine months in which she had made a good adjustment outside the hospital and was considered "remarkably improved." She had gained some insight into her condition by individual psychotherapy which had been supportive, too. It was felt, however, that the interest of the patient's family, especially the attitude of the patient's brother, who took her into his home and gave her a new goal and purpose in life, was of great importance in this patient's remission from her severe anxiety neurosis, complicated by hysterical and psychosomatic features.

CASE HISTORY NO. 2

This is the case history of a 59 year old male patient who became depressed and anxious because of sudden changes in his occupation which he believed were humiliating for him. He also became panicky because of financial difficulties which threatened his security.

He was treated by eight sessions of individual psychotherapy with the goal of gaining some insight into his condition, helping him to verbalize his hostility against his boss, giving him support and encouragement on a new job he disliked, keeping his self-esteem high, assisting him in recognizing his limitations in a realistic way, and making it possible for him to live without considering himself a burden for his family and superfluous. With the cooperation of the patient's wife, who was understanding and sympathetic, the individual psychotherpy was a success. The patient was able to adjust himself well on his changed job; he confronted his economical situation with a new emotional outlook and found a way toward a new life with serenity and fulfillment. *From the Outpatient Department of Galesburg State Research Hospital, November 1958.*

This patient was seen on an outpatient basis on the recommendation of his family physician. The patient was 59 years old, married, father of one boy who was graduated from college the year before, and of one girl who was graduated as a public health nurse, also the year before. Patient worked as a janitor and window washer at a power company since the previous September. Prior to this he held a job as a meter reader for about 10 years but was discharged because of decreased eyesight. The patient felt tired, down-hearted, unable to sleep, and was very slow in his work. He explained his attitude of not being able to do his present job because he was not "mechanically minded and never did a job like that." He also felt angry about a reduction in salary. Furthermore, he had debts amounting to about a thousand dollars to be paid on his new house. His wife suffered from a heart condition and took Digitalis daily. Although he felt down-hearted and suffered from crying spells occasionally, he did not think of suicide because "my religion does not permit it."

The patient was in good contact, oriented in all three spheres, his memory was fair for recent and remote events, and his intellectural capacities were of normal range. He was not interested, however, in reading newspapers any more and suffered from a certain apathy for the past couple of months. He was tense and anxious. His facial expression was one of depression and his whole attitude was one of hopelessness. He was cleanly dressed, wore eyeglasses which showed that he suffered from a rather serious myopia. He looked older than 59 years. He explained that he had suffered a heart attack in 1952. Ever since he was unable to do hard work.

Diagnostic Impression: Psychoneurosis with features of anxiety and depression, moderately severe, precipitated by his change of occupation.

Comments:

It appeared that the patient felt rather ashamed of his present status and suffered from an inferiority complex. He had felt humiliated and could not confront his son and daughter who had a higher education than he did. Individual psychotherapy was indicated. No tranqualizing drugs were ordered. The patient was seen on an outpatient basis, once weekly, for an hour.

Individual Psychotherapy Session 1

The patient returned in time for his first psychotherapy hour. He was tense and anxious and complained that he was unable to concentrate. He had felt himself "going to pieces" the day before. He cried "like a little boy" and believed that he would not be able to get up in the morning. Asked how he felt about coming to the therapy hour, he answered that he had no "pro or con feelings" but he did not resent it. He told his boss that he would get treatment by a psychiatrist. Then he continued to talk about his present job and how important it was for him to keep the job. But he had no interest in it. He used to be interested in politics but he did not read newspapers any more. Then he remarked that his wife suffered a heart attack the same morning. He felt very helpless. All he could do was to pray. He had no will power left. He lost faith in himself and could not sleep the night before. He complained that he did not like his present job because he was not used to "mechanical instruments." He mentioned that his boss always had been good to him and he did not understand why he had to do manual labor now. He expressed some hostility against his boss. At the end of the hour he said that he always had been a perfectionist and much concerned about himself. Now he was going through a "living hell." He also had a bad time as a child when his father and mother died. At the present he felt like wanting to die.

Individual Psychotherapy Sessions 2 and 3

The patient returned regularly for his outpatient appointment. On this day he was tense and frightened and said he would like to crawl into his bed and not get out any more. He had to force himself to do anything. His wife came at night to visit him on his job, brought him coffee and helped him to go on. He felt hopeless but forced himself to wash a couple of windows. He was avoiding seeing people. Before this demotion happened, they called him the "main street philosopher" but he did not feel like that now. His wife had asked him to sign a mortgage on his house in order to buy another house which was cheaper and did not need repairs. He was praying every day. It was a "torture" for him to go to work.

A week later the patient seemed much more relaxed and relieved. He still showed a compliant attitude, excused himself for not closing the door, stated that he took the psychiatrist's time but asked to smoke a cigarette and talked much more at ease. His main worry was the fact that he bought a new house but had not sold his old house yet and at this time he had two bills to pay for light and for other things for the new house which was still empty. He reproved himself that he did not sell his old house first before buying the other one. While he smoked a cigarette he remarked that he shouldn't smoke because he could not afford it. But he continued, "The Lord will help me." He did not despair any more. Then he said that he felt a certain amount of guilt because he had not been an "angel." He always tried to be a big shot, only he could not be one. At the end of the interview he said that he always liked to read adventure books and Westerns but had not done this for a long period of time. Now he felt like going to the library again.

Individual Psychotherapy Sessions 4 and 5

The patient returned punctually for his fourth outpatient appointment and immediately started to complain about his two houses which he "had on his neck." He was unable to sell one. Then he said that he read a book about the Korean War which he had at home but did not enjoy reading it. He tried to "analyze himself." He would like to know how much of his trouble was physical due to his age and how much was bad will. He believed he had signed the contract for his new house. Then he talked about his boy who changed his job. He was now on the personnel staff of a college. He remarked that he went shopping but avoided meeting people. At the end of the interview he was more cheerful and started to smile. He made the remark that although he was worried, he did not worry about his funeral yet.

At the next meeting, he looked more relaxed. He mentioned having "nervous spells" at home but he could hardly wait to come to his therapy hour because "the therapist was so understanding." Again he talked about his houses and said that he couldn't figure things out. However, he was getting along better with his work, nobody complained about him or said anything negative. He remarked that he smoked two packs of cigarettes a day and felt that was too much. He could do better things with the money than spending it on cigarettes; he could go to a movie once in a while. He read a new book, *The Robe*. He liked it very much. Then he spoke about his job. He did not like the physical effort in connection with it but did not want to quit because he would be getting a pension.

He went the previous Sunday to another town to see his son-in-law. He watched a movie on television about a treasure buried during the Civil War in New Orleans. He went away relaxed and in a good mood.

Individual Psychotherapy Sessions 6 and 7

The patient returned for outpatient psychotherapy the following week. He remarked that he had nice holidays, watching television and attending church. He still did not feel completely relaxed. Then he talked about his experiences as a "house servant" in Germany after World War I. He liked the atmosphere of his job and got a lot out of it. He never wanted to be quite dependent but liked to stay employed. Then he spoke about a heart attack he suffered in 1952, together with pneumonia. He bought only one new suit of clothes since he married. He did not like to spend money but thought he now spent too much for cigarettes. He realized that changes upset him and that he had difficulties with "technical advances." He thought he made friends easily and would have been very good in "public relations." He did not like jazz music but preferred "good music" only.

The patient returned the following week and appeared relaxed, more secure of himself and in a better mood. He read some books and watched television. He spoke about the Americans treating minorities badly and how unjust this was. He then made remarks about consumers and production and went on talking about political matters of the day.

Comment:

It appeared that he wanted to impress the therapist with his general knowledge about politics. The patient apparently had overcome his depression. He was much better adjusted on his present job. The therapist talked to the patient's wife who was waiting, and encouraged her to have patience. She left in a hopeful mood.

Individual Psychotherapy Session 8

The patient returned the following week. He saw books on Aging on my desk and remarked, "That's for me. I felt it during the last few months." He was less tense. He stated that he had 4 people interested in buying his old house but his wife agreed now that they had been hasty in buying the new house. Then he told about a book he read about Buffalo Bill. He was the last of the great scouts and killed 40,000 buffaloes. He continued saying he could not complain too much and that he was "back to normal" again. His aspect was one of a man looking younger than he had looked; the features of depression were gone.

He was proud that his son was elected to the staff alumni association of a college. He said that once he met the mental health director at the same college at a private party. Both his son and the director's son were students. He said that the only difference between the director of mental health and himself was "I have no money." Then he laughed.

Comment:

The patient had completely recovered from his features of depression and anxiety and was released from psychotherapy; he was told to return to the hospital and get an appointment at some future time if needed. He did not return. His wife let us know six months later that he was well adjusted on his new job and "felt fine."

A SODIUM AMYTAL INTERVIEW
December 1955

This is a Sodium Amytal interview of a 75 year old patient who suffered from a Chronic Brain Syndrome, associated with Senility, moderate, with features of a neurotic depression. The patient improved with group psychotherapy for three months. He was transferred to an "exit ward" but fell down and received a fracture of his leg. He again became depressed, refused to eat and was uncommunicative. With his own permission, a Sodium Amytal interview was given to him, of about 20 minutes' duration, to find out the psychological cause of his depression. It was suspected that he felt ambivalent about staying at the hospital or leaving it. He would have to take care of himself but considered living with his son.

The Sodium Amytal interview was given in the presence of the head nurse and nurse in charge of the ward:

Doctor: What happened to you? How did you fall?

Patient: I was on the ward. I broke my leg and they sent me to Kansas City and then they brought me back. They had me in a cast for a while.

Doctor: How did it happen that you broke your leg?

Patient: Well, sir, it seems awfully silly. You know they have rollers on the legs of the beds and some of the rollers have brakes on them and some of them don't. Well, sometimes they are not put on and the bed will roll. One night I got up and wanted to go to the bathroom. I reached under the bed to get my house shoes and the brakes were not set and I slipped out and broke my leg.

Doctor: When did you come back to this hospital?

Patient: I don't remember. Time flies.

Doctor: Why did you come back?

Patient: I don't know. They sent me.

Doctor: Did you drink?

Patient: Yes, sir, a little bit. That was years ago. I do not drink to excess.

Doctor: How long ago was that?

Patient: Oh, I would say about 10 years ago. It seems about that long.

Doctor: Why did you start? Were you unhappy about something?
Patient: Oh, I just drank socially.
Doctor: Could you not stop?
Patient: I did.
Doctor: But, Mr. ———, why did you come back here to the hospital?
Patient: I got sick and came back. I came back because I wanted to. I was here before and I had no place else to go. I could not afford to go to a private clinic.
Doctor: Why did you not go home?
Patient: I have no home.
Doctor: Who took care of you before you came here?
Patient: I took care of myself.
Doctor: How did you feel about that?
Patient: Oh, I worried about things—money and things.
Doctor: You lived alone?
Patient: Yes, my wife died in 1935.
Doctor: Do you have any children?
Patient: Yes, I have a son and a daughter. My daughter died.
Doctor: Why don't you go to your son?
Patient: They don't want me. They have a nice home but my daughter-in-law does not want anyone to live with them. She would not let her own father live with them.
Doctor: Why does she not want a nice gentleman like you?
Patient: I don't know. She is just that way.
Doctor: Does your daughter-in-law not like you?
Patient: I don't think so.
Doctor: What does your son do?
Patient: He works for a creamery.
Doctor: Does he earn good money?
Patient: Oh, no. They have bought a new home. They bought it "on time;" he still has to pay for it.
Doctor: Do you have only one son?
Patient: That is right.
Doctor: When you fell in the other building, did they want to send you out of the hospital?
Patient: (Did not answer.)
Doctor: Were you excited or nervous?

Patient: No, I got along well.
Doctor: Why can't you live on the outside?
Patient: I don't have enough money. I only get $75 a month.
Doctor: You can't live on that?
Patient: No, sir.
Doctor: How much rent do you pay?
Patient: I paid $20 a month. I got along well, but I got sick. I wasn't myself, and so I told my son to bring me here.
Doctor: What should we do here to help you?
Patient: Get me perfectly well and walking. I'd like to go home again.
Doctor: What would you do at home?
Patient: I would cook and eat and live.
Doctor: Have you always been alone?
Patient: No, I was married.
Doctor: Do you miss your wife very much?
Patient: Very much! She was a fine woman, a very good woman. We lived together a great number of years.
Doctor: Were you always happy?
Patient: Very happy.
Doctor: What happened to your daughter?
Patient: She died of a gunshot wound. She committed suicide. My wife died of cancer and my daughter lived with the fear she would have it.
Doctor: Did she get it?
Patient: No.
Doctor: Was your daughter married?
Patient: No.
Doctor: Did you ever think of killing yourself?
Patient: Oh, no. I want to live. Even here I am not too unhappy.
Doctor: What can we do to make you happier?
Patient: I can't think of anything. I would like to get rid of the pain in my leg.
Doctor: What was your occupation before you came to the hospital?
Patient: I used to be a cook. I was a very good chef. I worked many years.
Doctor: How did your health get bad?

Patient: Oh, it was not my heart. Cooking is unhealthy after a time. After I worked for a cement company I bought a restaurant. I couldn't get enough help. I worked too hard and I got sick.

Doctor: Where is the restaurant? Did you sell it?

Patient: Yes, I got sick and had to sell.

Doctor: Why did you come to this hospital? Don't you know this is a hospital for "mental" patients?

Patient: Yes. There is nothing wrong with my mind. It is pretty good, you will have to admit that.

Doctor: Is your son interested in you?

Patient: I think he is interested, but he does not want to keep me. They have a little girl taking piano lessons and a nice home. My daughter-in-law does not want her own father there.

Doctor: Do you have any friends?

Patient: I suppose so.

Doctor: Why do you not go to stay with your friends?

Patient: Oh, you don't go to friends. I would not ask them to do anything for me.

Doctor: Are you too proud?

Patient: I seem to be. I have always been a good man and lived clean.

Doctor: You say you have lived a clean life. Did you drink?

Patient: A little bit.

Doctor: Have you been drunk?

Patient: I have been a little tight, but never drunk.

Doctor: Did you go to church?

Patient: Yes.

Doctor: Did you ever commit any crime?

Patient: No, I never committed any crime at all. I have always meant well to other people.

Doctor: What about your daughter-in-law? Do you like her?

Patient: Yes, I like her.

Doctor: Are you sure?

Patient: Absolutely.

Doctor: Do you think your son is a good son?

Patient: He is a fine son. A good boy.

Doctor: When did your wife die?
Patient: In 1935.
Doctor: How did you feel?
Patient: Very badly.
Doctor: Did you ever consider marrying again?
Patient: I thought about it, but my fiancee died.
Doctor: How long ago was that?
Patient: Three years ago.
Doctor: How old was she?
Patient: She was not young. She was 60. She ran a store and did very well. She was a very efficient woman.
Doctor: What did she die of?
Patient: She died of a heart condition.
Doctor: What about your future?
Patient: I'll wait and see how I come out. I want to get well and not be crippled up.
Doctor: Do you feel lonesome?
Patient: Yes, sometimes.
Doctor: If you get well, what will you do then?
Patient: I'll try to go home again. I am just so short on money. I got behind, but I am paying to catch up. I am paying to the state. I feel I owe it.
Doctor: Were you a good worker?
Patient: All my life.
Doctor: Did you ever want to die before your wife died?
Patient: No, I wanted to live.
Doctor: If you live 20 years more, what would you like to do?
Patient: I don't know. I am too old to do anything. I am 75 years old. Nobody wants a 75 year old man. You will find that out when you reach that age.
Doctor: What do you think of a nursing home?
Patient: I do not think I have enough money to do anything.
Doctor: Do you need treatment for your mind?
Patient: No, sir. There is not a damned thing wrong with my mind.
Doctor: Other people thought so, didn't they?
Patient: Well, they are wrong.

Comment:

The Welfare Department of the State was advised about the patient's condition and checked into his and his son's financial condition. It was decided to have him transferred to a nursing home where Public Welfare would pay full maintenance. The patient left the hospital after two months when he was able to move around. Successful surgery was performed for his leg fracture. The patient's progress in the nursing home was carefully checked. He adjusted well and was not in need of further help from the hospital. His depression subsided completely when he became interested in another "nice lady" at the nursing home.

B. GROUP PSYCHOTHERAPY

Group psychotherapy was attempted with geriatric patients by Silver (141) for the first time in 1950. His group psychotherapy was part of an integrated treatment program for female patients between the ages of 70 and 80 years. This new kind of therapy, according to Silver, improved not only the morale of the patients but also of the nurses. It heartened and thereby furthered the cooperation of the relatives who recognized that, at last, active treatment was being given to the elderly patients. Silver had some difficulty in handling the reiteration by certain patients of specific topics. He eventually developed a special interviewing technique to guide the group toward other topics. Among these overly-discussed topics were:

1. The "good old days,"
2. Social and economic difficulties,
3. Feelings of rejection by one's own family,
4. Complaints about the routine on the ward,
5. The loneliness of old age,
6. Physical ailments.

Schwartz and Goodman (131) used group psychotherapy with obese elderly diabetics in 1952. Of 19 patients, only 6 remained overweight at the end of the treatment. Two of the 19 patients were able to discontinue their insulin. These patients were considered "hopeless" before group psychotherapy.

S. Benaim (11) treated 18 male geriatric patients in groups of 7 to 10 patients at the Geriatric Unit at Bethlehem Royal Hospital for a period of three to four months. The patients received group psychotherapy once a week for one hour and a half. The average age of the members was 68 years. Benaim reported good results and felt that this technique definitely helped his patients toward a better adjustment to the hospital environment.

A more controlled and extensive study has been made by M. Linden (105, 108) at the Norristown State Hospital in Pennsylvania. Linden treated a group of 51 women whose average age was over 70. Treatment extended for a few years with the group meeting twice weekly for one hour sessions. Most of these patients took part in these sessions regularly. A special effort was made to encourage free association, uninhibited verbalization and mutual interpretation. After six months of relatively unpromising results, a nurse was introduced as co-leader of the group. Better group identity occurred, and finally, during the eighth and ninth months of treatment, many members of the group became more alert, took greater interest in occupational and recreational activities. Feminine identification with the co-leader was enhanced and transference toward the male, protective, parental therapist was increased. The atmosphere of pessimism and inactivity diminished. Of this group, 23 left the hospital for their own homes, county homes or foster homes, or were felt ready to leave after an average of 54 hours of group psychotherapy. Linden used a control group of 279 other geriatric patients who did not receive group psychotherapy. Only 27 of these were released from the hospital. To be noted are Linden's techniques which included didactic talks to stimulate his group members, individual questioning concerning biographical data, and, at times, treatment of his patients with good-natured sarcasm.

My own experience with group psychotherapy for geriatric patients dates back to September 1954 when group psychotherapy was started in a geriatric unit of a Kansas state hospital affiliated with the Menninger Foundation. Since then, I have continued this form of treatment with geriatric groups at the State Research Hospital in Galesburg (Illinois), for a period of one year, and, finally, for two and a half years at the Veterans Administration Hospital in Coatesville (Pennsylvania).

My observations and studies made with group psychotherapy and its significance for Geriatric Psychiatry have been published on different occasions (152, 157, 158). Group psychotherapy should be an important part of the treatment program for the geriatric patient in a psychiatric institution. My technique is different from Linden's and involves both male and female patients. Since 1954, my groups have been composed of three or four men and three or four women. Fruit juice and cigarettes are offered, and the patients are encouraged to serve themselves and to talk about their problems in an informal way. The therapist introduces the members to one another. The reason for the meetings, they are told, is for them to come together to become friends, to help one another, and to learn about one another's problems. Criticism of the therapist himself, of the nurses and attendants, of the meals and the hospital methods and organization is encouraged. The attitude of the therapist is a passive one. He merely listens to the patients and interferes only on rare occasions when one patient or another is mute and has to be encouraged to take active part in the conversation. The therapist is considered to be an understanding brother who answers questions when they are of general interest to the group, but who occasionally has to discourage questions which interest single members only and can be answered in his office privately. The therapist sometimes turns questions and problems back to the other members of the group.

Criteria of Selection

The patients are selected after careful consideration of their physical and mental condition. The criteria are chosen by the therapist, according to the goal he has in mind. In the geriatric group, patients with too many physical complaints or serious illnesses are excluded because of the possibility of sudden death or chronic sickness which might make them bedfast. Those chosen are able to hear fairly well and to see those with whom they talk. They do not talk in a confused way. They are in fairly good contact with their surroundings, are not overly psychotic, and do not suffer from delusions or hallucinations which take all of their attention. There are no signs of a progressive deterioration of their intellectual faculties and memory.

They can, however, show signs of partial disorientation, a slightly impaired memory for recent events, retardation of psychomotor activity, as long as they are not completely mute. They can be hostile and express delusional material, as long as they are at times in contact with reality or are felt to have the potentiality to regain contact. If they reveal signs of restlessness and anxiety, they are still accepted, unless they are so restless that they pace the office during the meeting. Seclusive patients are welcome. It makes no difference whether the patients are psychotic or neurotic with some senile or arteriosclerotic changes. It was necessary, however, that those chosen for group psychotherapy had the possibility for improvement.

During a period of 6 years, in three different psychiatric hospitals, 110 geriatric patients were treated by this form of group psychotherapy. The sessions were of 50 minutes' duration, once a week. The average age of the patients was 63 years. The majority of these patients belonged to the schizophrenic group (70%) and they had been hospitalized for an average time of 20 years. Twenty-five percent included patients suffering from a mild to moderate chronic brain syndrome associated with cerebral arteriosclerosis or senility. Three percent were diagnosed as suffering from chronic brain syndrome associated with syphilis; and two percent with chronic alcoholism. Of these 110 geriatric patients, 40 were females. All patients were evaluated prior to the beginning of the group psychotherapy sessions by psychiatric examination and psychological testing, which was repeated at six-month intervals.

Geriatric patients are very conservative, sensitive and emotional. At times they show an attitude of rigidity and inflexibility with compulsive and overtly moralistic trends. Such behavior, whenever observed, appeared to be a sign of decompensation—a desperate trial to hold the personality together, a fight against desperation, against the feelings of complete confusion and fear of being lost. When a patient showed improvement, these symptoms disappeared and were replaced by the ability to relax and by decreased rigidity.

Thought Content of the Patients

Very interesting studies could be made in regard to the thought content. The most frequent topics chosen for discussion by members of the group were:

1. Religion,
2. Marriage and love life,
3. Historical events, and
4. Food.

Religion was the preferred topic of the members of the group. Unhappy, lonesome and despondent patients were eager to discuss a better life after death, in paradise, perceived by them as a heaven of love and kindness. The religious attitude increased when the personality disintegrated and became disorganized. Religious belief, faith in God, helped them to overcome their grief. The other members of the group hardly ever doubted such a religious trend, because religion gave to all of them support and greater Ego strength. Delusions of religion were not infrequent. Some of the patients suffered from visual or auditory hallucinations, believing that they heard the voice of the Lord or that they saw Him. However, whenever a patient expressed delusions of persecution, of being mistreated by friends or relatives, his words were not accepted by the other members of the group as true and correct, and the possibility of a mistake or a wrong interpretation of the relative's words or actions was discussed. Delusions of grandeur were even less accepted. When a member of the group believed himself to be very rich, to own factories or houses, or to be a good friend of the governor or another politician, he was openly doubted. This attitude had the effect, after initial irritability and resentment, of bringing the delusional patient nearer to reality.

Nearly all patients expressed deep attachment to their spouse. They showed anger against them only during the acute phase of their sickness. Hostility toward their children was a more frequent topic for discussion. Resentment, disappointment, hate, feelings of being rejected and a burden to the younger generation were ventilated. They felt somewhat relieved in knowing that other members of the group had suffered troubles of a similar kind. Thus they came closer to one another and their interpersonal relationships improved remarkably. It was common for widowed patients to reflect upon the good things experienced in the past and to share these with the group. Many of them did not believe, at the beginning of the group meetings, that the dead partner could ever be substituted. Erotic feelings were repressed at first, but, after a couple of months, the men and women looked at each other with affection. They started to dress with more care. The men shaved more regularly, came to the meetings with their best ties and washed themselves more frequently. The ladies began to use lipstick and to powder their faces. This change in the patients' attitudes toward their personal appearance was one of the first, and perhaps the most important good response to group psychotherapy. The socialization and rehabilitation process was enhanced and interest in marriage and love did reappear.

Some of the patients, irritated at first by the presence of members of the opposite sex, gradually lost their suspicion, showed more interest, and became friendlier. When a member of the group fell sick, the others visited him in the infirmary ward or sent get-well cards. Couples who sat side by side during the group therapy session were also seen together at the dances, at movies, at birthday parties, and at other occupational or recreational activities.

Another subject of conversation chosen very often was historical events. They liked to talk about kings and queens of the countries of their families' origin, about the early settlements in the United States, about religious and political customs of fifty or more years ago, about the Indians, the Spanish-American War, and about famous American poets and artists. Technical progress —cars, the use of phones, modern machinery and farm equipment —were rarely brought into the conversation.

They liked to read books about the Civil War in the United States and showed a rather conservative inclination toward the problem of racial discrimination. At times they were not very tolerant. They appeared to be threatened by revolutionary ideas and occasionally showed ambivalent feelings toward new immigrants. Newcomers not speaking good English were initially not easily accepted, but, as time went on, they found better understanding and sympathy and formed friendships with the other participants of the group.

Unless physically sick, geriatric patients like to eat and show a certain amount of regression to the oral stage. Consequently, one of the most important topics of discussion during the meeting was food. Candies and chocolates were exchanged. The meals on holidays and birthday parties which included cookies and cakes were very often mentioned. Stomach trouble, because of overeating, was a frequent event.

For elderly patients, too great a preoccupation with eating or digestive problems is not a favorable symptom. It can be considered as a regression into infantile, immature, and dependent behavior which might be reinforced by an overprotective attitude of relatives or attendants. For some patients, this kind of regression into excessive oral cravings might become a serious handicap to their treatment and to their release from the hospital.

Group psychotherapy with geriatric patients at the Coatesville Veterans Administration Hospital was started in 1958 and has continued ever since. The veterans in my group sessions at this hospital were relatively less shy, less seclusive and less embarrassed. They revealed less difficulty in talking and relating to members of the other sex. They were relatively better groomed and well nourished and showed greater self-confidence. Generally, they felt less lonesome and rejected.

They had a better understanding of what was going on outside the hospital.

For the elderly patients in state mental hospitals, religion, marriage, love life, historical events and food were the most frequent topics of discussion. However, the veterans of this study were more interested in daily political events and in the current economic situation. Most of them read the newspaper daily and watched television. At times they distorted political facts and misinterpreted economic conditions. On these occasions they would get angry and excited and ventilate hostility. Frequently they tried to rationalize their own feelings of insecurity by considering themselves victims of unfortunate circumstances and believed they were justified in finding and asking for protection at all times.

One of the most noteworthy features of our patients was that they were proud to be veterans. They implied that all nonveterans owed them respect and gratitude. They expected special consideration and privileges.

Money and possessions were of extreme value to the veterans

and represented security to them. Religious problems were discussed frequently, showing their strong concern with life after death. However, the general attitude was one of apathy and disinterest when other persons were involved.

A further characteristic attitude was their conservatism and their resistance against any changes. They even resented a change from a closed to an open ward where they could enjoy more freedom of movement. Changes in recreation or in industrial therapy assignments were not welcomed. Changes of places in the dining room were opposed. New physicians or new nursing personnel were regarded with distrust. They did, however, keep close ties with their own families who considered them not much of a burden.

In connection with their resistance against changes, most of our patients lacked motivation to return to their family and community life. They thought themselves surrounded by a hostile world without empathy and pity and were afraid to try and adjust themselves outside the hospital again and to look for employment.

Results:

Of the 110 patients of the elderly age group treated by group psychotherapy, 40% showed improvement and were released from hospitalization. The improvement became evident three months after the group sessions were started. Generally, six months of treatment were necessary to secure a better emotional equilibrium. About 10% of the patients needed more than six months but less than one year before they were released from hospitalization. The first signs of improvement became evident in their improved grooming and eating habits. The patients started to verbalize their feelings, were able to control their hostility better and made a better ward adjustment. They started to communicate with one another more than before, made friends and took part in occupational and recreational activities together. Some of the patients who had been confused and out of contact at times, now talked more coherently. Others lost their paranoid ideas which they had expressed occasionally. Criticism by other members of the group, and doubts about their persecutory delusions helped them to come nearer reality.

According to my observation, the sex of the patient did not make any difference with regard to improvement. However, group psychotherapy given to geriatric patients of both sexes was definitely of greater curative effect than that given to control groups with only male patients. The increased interest of male and female patients in each other, the formation of friendships between them, the verbalization of motherly feelings of the women toward the men, and the protective attitude of the male patients toward the females had a remarkably therapeutic advantage. Other control groups, comprising patients who were treated by occupational or recreational activities alone, without group therapy, revealed the superior value of group psychotherapy with geriatric patients as a therapeutic tool. The improvement of patients in these control groups was of a minor degree only. Follow-ups were done after six months and one year and confirmed the stability of the patients' improvements by group psychotherapy which made it possible for them to adjust outside the hospital. Only two patients returned, after their release from hospitalization, for additional group pyschotherapy sessions once a week for the duration of four months. After that period of time, they were not in need of them any more.

Goals and Limitations of Group Psychotherapy with Geriatric Patients

According to my own experience, group psychotherapy for elderly patients is to be preferred over individual psychotherapy because it is less alarming to elderly patients than talking to the therapist in an individual session. Anxiety is decreased in group psychotherapy, transference to one or more members of the group is easier to achieve because of the variety of choices, and meaningful discussions are possible because a common goal or interest can be found with less effort. In this way the interpersonal relationships can improve quickly and with less resistance. In a group of geriatric patients, a patient who tends to distort the therapist into a fear-inspiring figure, feels the presence of others to be a protection for him. Acceptance by the group is at times more important to a patient than acceptance by an individual. Furthermore, feelings of difference and isolation decrease because the patients' problems are shared by others. The group may also be stimulating for the patient who must compete for the interest of the therapist and struggle for status in the group where he is brought into contact among persons of different background and outlook.

Most important, however, is the fact that the geriatric patient is encouraged to express his feelings in the group, that he has to clarify his ideas and has to respond to the attitude of others. In this way, the delusional elderly patient is forced to face the facts of reality and might be exposed to disapproval of the group. Feelings of being neglected or discriminated against by the younger generation might be criticized by other members of the group if these feelings do not actually appear to be justified. Frequently the patients in my group did correct other members expressing delusions of grandeur without antagonizing them. In this way, a more realistic outlook on life for elderly citizens is achieved by common effort and group interaction, a process much more difficult to promote in individual sessions. Observing also the usually liberal and generally relaxed attitude of other patients in the geriatric group discussing their problems openly, helps the patients to overcome their fear of the hated authority figure of the doctor or hostility against competing siblings which may represent one of their greatest problems. In this way, hostility is verbalized and decreased.

Finally, each member of the group is helped to grow toward a higher level of emotional maturity. Negative transference in the geriatric group becomes apparent at times between single members of the group and the therapist, or between members of the group thmselves. Countertransference phenomena might become of great concern for the therapist who does not like a patient reminding him of his own father or of an important figure of his past life, producing hostility in him. Such countertransference phenomena might thus become an obstacle in the way of therapeutic progress. The problem of identification is also of great importance in geriatric group psychotherapy. If members of the group are able to identify with others in the group, this event would be beneficial, influencing the whole atmosphere of the group. When the therapist is able and willing to identify with his group, this, too, represents a great advantage. For this purpose, the therapist for a geriatric group shoud not be too old or too young and should be in good emotional equilibrium himself. The therapist should convey, most of all, empathy and hope to his patients and be convinced that he is able to help them.

Another much-discussed problem in regard to group psychotherapy with geriatric patients and its therapeutic aim is the gaining of insight. Some insight can be achieved through group psychotherapy. Other therapists are inclined to emphasize less the process of gaining insight than of resocialization and the return to a higher degree of self-sufficiency (Linden, Benaim). According to my experience, the development of deep insight for elderly citizens is frequently not only impossible but also undesirable. Geriatric patients reveal, at times, a certain inflexibility of character and attitude, due to increasing age, which is one of their basic characteristics and which is difficult to change. They also suffer often from impaired memory as part of a brain damage due to pathological changes in the brain substance itself and really forget some important events of their lives. Other problems, involving insomnia and restlessness, fear of closing their eyes at night and feelings of being frightened in the dark, so frequent in elderly persons, need to be handled with great skill and circumspection. According to my own observations, these symptoms of insomnia and restless agitation are expressions of their fear of dying and their ambivalent feelings toward life and death. Letting elderly patients gain insight into this specific condition might disturb them greatly and can increase their symptoms. Support, rather than insight, is indicated and is more helpful on such occasions.

I believe, however, that group psychotherapy is of definite usefulness to geriatric patients when the focus is placed on increasing socialization, interpersonal relationships and group identity, and encouraging self-expression. Repair of the underlying personality conflicts is possible and advisable in only limited ways.

C. SOMATIC THERAPIES

Research projects and clinical observations on the use of drugs for emotionally disturbed geriatric patients are many. The results obtained are frequently contradictory. When psychopharmacological drugs were introduced in the United States around 1954, the opinion of psychiatrists differed according to training and background. Psychoanalysts and psychoanalytically oriented psychiatrists saw a danger in handling emotional disturbances by other than psychological means and preferred psychotherapy and milieutherapy. Psychiatrists with an inclination to handle emotional problems by biological methods, lobotomies, electric shock treatment or insulin coma, believed that the new drugs would become an important therapeutic tool. Some of them believed the time was coming when the cause of schizophrenia and other mental sicknesses would be discovered in faulty metabolism of the brain and the central nervous system or in defects of the blood or circulatory system. These biologically oriented psychiatrists favored treatment with drugs and minimized the importance of a psychodynamic approach in the treatment of the mental patient.

At the present time, after more than seven years of experiments with psychopharmacological drugs in the United States, the majority of psychiatrists believe that these medications make patients more approachable to psychiatric treatment generally. Indeed the treatment of the psychotically disturbed, excited, delusional and hostile patient; of the apathetic, listless and regressed schizophrenic; and of the deeply depressed, suicidal patient has improved considerably through the use of the modern psychopharmacological drugs.

I remember well my frustrations and disappointments before psychopharmacological drugs were given. For hostile, threatening and excited psychotic and non-psychotic patients, the drugs of choice were sedatives and hypnotics.

These drugs did not make the patients more approachable to psychotherapy of any kind. They felt dizzy and drowsy after the use of them and became disturbed when the effect of the medication wore off. Elderly patients, on the morning after having received sedative medication, stumbled, often fell down and suffered fractures.

There is no doubt in my mind that the modern psychopharmacological drugs are particularly useful because they do not produce marked feelings of drowsiness but quiet the excited and disturbed patients and help them toward a better adjustment to the hospital and finally to accept psychiatric treatment.

The literature on psychopharmacological drugs is tremendous and growing continuously. For this reason it would be impossible to describe all of the results obtained from experiments and studies of geriatric psychiatric chemotherapy. As soon as such a book or paper is published, the observations described might already be outdated. Therefore, I will be able to report only my own experiences collected through a period of over seven years of treating elderly patients in psychiatric institutions. My results are of a subjective nature only and might not be confirmed by results obtained by other gerontologists or psychiatrists. They are, however, in most instances, obtained from controlled studies. Frequenty double-blind methods were used. On other occasions the patients were evaluated by psychiatric, neurological and physical examination before, during and after the experiments. Psychological testing was always given in order to get more objective results. There is no foreseeable end or limit to be set for further experiments with drugs for the emotionally disturbed geriatric patient. New, more effective and less toxic psychopharmacological drugs will inevitably be developed.

I. Psychopharmacological Drugs Used for Agitated, Excited, Tense and Hostile Geriatric Patients

In different psychiatric hospitals since 1954, I have had experience with chlorpromazine (Thorazine), reserpine (Serpasil), promazine hydrochloride (Sparine), mepazine (Pacatal), meprobamate (Miltown), perphenazine (Trilafon), Prochlorperazine (Compazine), Trifluoperazine (Stelazine), methaminodiazepoxide (Librium), thioridazine (Mellaril), and others. According to my own observations, chlorpromazine is to be considered an effective drug which did show, in most instances, results in two to three weeks after the beginning of the medication. For most patients, the maximum effect occurred after three months of drug administration. The results became more or less stabilized after that time. Generally, disturbed and agitated geriatric patients became quieter and more cooperative and could be reached during or after this period of time by group- or individual psychotherapy or milieutherapy. The average dosage used was 50 mg., three times daily. In rare cases more than 200 mg. of chlorpromazine were found to be needed by elderly patients. Side effects occurred in less than 2% of my patients and decreased when the dosage of the medication was decreased or the drug discontinued. Hypotension was observed rather early in treatment in 1% of my patients. Shock reaction occurred rarely. Dry mouth and nasal congestion and blurred vision were observed in 2% of my cases. Intrahepatic obstructive jaundice, agranulocytosis and neutropenia and the Parkinson syndrome with signs of rigidity, tremor, increased salivation were seen in about 1% of my patients. Severe depressions with chlorpromazine were observed only in 1 case out of 500 patients treated with this drug. There was essentially no difference in regard to results or toxic effects for men or women. The drug was given to more than 1000 geriatric patients, under my supervision, since 1954. The ages varied from 60 to 91 years. The diagnoses of the agitated geriatric patients varied from Schizophrenic Reaction to Acute or Chronic Brain Syndromes, associated with various causes (Alcoholism, Lues of the brain, Cerebral Arteriosclerosis, Senility). Among the other tranquilizing medications, thioridazine (Mellaril) would be my second choice in regard to effectiveness. The side effects of thioridazine seemed to be lesser (observation on 200 patients) than of chlorpromazine. Meprobamate is to be preferred for elderly patients with psychoneurotic disorders. This drug made it possible for excited patients of this kind to start individual or group psychotherapy after a period of one week.

The results obtained by phenothiazine derivatives like chlorpromazine and thioridazine are explained by their effect upon subcortical action: stimulating the amygdaloid complex, depression of the hypothalamus and the reticular activating system. Emotional response to external and internal stimuli is diminished and the patients become less excited and anxious.

While insulin shock treatment for geriatric patients has been found risky due to disturbances of liver function, insulin subcoma treatment has been found useful and effective previous to the use of tranquilizing medication. The patients suffering from tenseness and restless, agitated behavior were treated with up to 70 units of regular insulin injections early in the morning. After two to three hours they got drowsy and sleepy and eventually started to perspire slightly. The patients then were fed with fruit juice containing sugar and recovered after four hours from their drowsy and sleepy condition completely. This method was used by myself successfully for more than 40 geriatric patients of various diagnoses. It was given daily, five days weekly, for four weeks. Seventy-five percent of the patients became quieter and more cooperative. I abandoned subcoma insulin treatment, however, after the use of the psychopharmacological drugs became known and showed satisfactory results. The reason for abandoning this form of treatment was more of an administrative nature because insulin subcoma treatment required more extensive nursing care and supervision. It was also found to be more expensive.

II. Psychopharmacological Drugs for Depressed Geriatric Patients

Since 1956 I have treated more than 150 geriatric patients with antidepressive drugs and have been able to observe the effectiveness of some of them.

My experience with antidepressive drugs for geriatric patients up to the present is restricted to studies made with iproniazid (Marsilid), phenelzine (Nardil), nialamide (Niamid), and imipramine (Tofranil). The first three drugs represent monoamine oxidase inhibitors. A study made at a Kansas state hospital with 30 geriatric patients who were treated with iproniazid in a dosage of 50 mg., twice daily, was discontinued after three weeks. Four patients suffered from severe agitation with relapse into their delusional system. It caused moderate improvement, however, in 6 of my 30 geriatric patients suffering from features of a psychotic depression. This improvement took place after three weeks of the use of this medication.

Nialamide had been used successfully for 32 patients of ages 58 to 61. They suffered from involutional depression. Of these 32 patients, 15 showed lessening of their depressive symptoms after a period of 4 weeks. Nialamide was given in dosage of 100 mg., twice daily.

Imipramine was used for 34 geriatric patients ranging in age from 59 to 70 years. Four of them were diagnosed as psychotic depression, 17 as Chronic Brain Syndrome, associated with Cerebral Arteriosclerosis, 13 as Senility with neurotic depression. The dosage given was 100 mg., daily for four weeks. Nineteen improved moderately and made a better ward adjustment. However, 4 of them relapsed into their depressive state two days after the drug was discontinued. Side effects were noted in 3 of the 34 patients during the second week. They suffered from increased agitation and insomnia. When the dosage was decreased for them, the toxic effects subsided.

Phenelzine in dosage of 45 mg. daily was given to another group of 30 geriatric patients with an average age of 67 years. Of these, 14 were diagnosed as Chronic Brain Syndrome, associated with Cerebral Arteriosclerosis, and 16 were diagnosed as Senility with psychotic depression. For these patients, electric shock treatment could not be given due to their weakened physical condition. These patients suffered from severe arthritic changes of their vertebral column or had a history of myocardial infarction. Seventeen improved slightly after 5 weeks of medication and continued to hold their improvement. Side effects were not observed.

My studies made with antidepressive medication did not compare favorably, however, with the application of electric shock treatment in the psychotically depressed and suicidal geriatric patient. Four electric shock treatments, given twice weekly, were of greater benefit. Of 36 geriatric patients treated with electric shock, 25 improved remarkably after four treatments and lost their suicidal tendencies. These patients, after a period of one additional month, could be treated by milieutherapy and group psychotherapy and were released in less than four months from hospitalization.

III. Psychopharmacological Drugs Used for Withdrawn and Apathetic Geriatric Patients

Although Stelazine (trifluoperazine) belongs to the group of tranquilizing medication, my own observations found this drug useful and indicated for withdrawn, seclusive, listless and apathetic geriatric patients suffering from Chronic Brain Syndrome associated with Senility, Arteriosclerosis, or from Schizophrenic Reaction, Chronic Undifferentiated Type. These patients belonged to the group of idle patients who needed to be motivated to participate in ward or other activities and were very resistant. They were not interested in anything and, left to their own devices, regressed further and became more uncommunicative. Twenty-four of my patients were treated with trifluoperazine, belonging to the age group of 60 to 81 years. Ten were females and 14 were males. The average dosage was 6 mg., twice daily. Side effects observed in 2 of these patients were drowsiness and Parkinsonism which became evident after 4 weeks of use of the drug. Of these 24 patients, only 6 improved moderately while 2 improved only slightly after 4 weeks of medication. They became more interested in activities on the ward and more talkative.

At the Veterans Administration Hospital at Coatesville (Pa.) in 1959, a controlled study with Nialamide for 20 chronic elderly schizophrenic male patients was made. (161) The mean age of the group was 60 years, 3 months. The mean length of hospitalization was 24 years, 8 months. The initial dosage of Nialamide (Niamid) was 25 mg., twice daily. After one month the dosage was increased to 25 mg., 1 tablet t.i.d. Following this dosage, and after three weeks' duration, Niamid 25 mg., 6 tablets daily (150 mg.) were given. This dosage, after three additional weeks, was increased for the duration of 22 days to 8 tablets, 25 mg. each, daily (200 mg.). After 22 days of treatment with this final dosage, the treatment was discontinued.

This study indicated that after the end of the three-month period of medication, one patient was moderately improved. He became more talkative, more alert, more relaxed and was in better contact. Six patients were improved slightly. They became more alert, more talkative, more cooperative and showed increased interest in activities. Eleven patients did not show any change. Two patients became worse. One of these became more hostile and delusional to a moderate degree. The same patient's physical condition showed a change for the worse and, being underweight, he lost two pounds in weight. One patient became slightly worse. He, too, showed increased agitation and hostility. His physical condition remained unchanged. Two patients revealed side effects after three months of medication (dryness of tongue and of the lips). No other side effects had been observed.

The improvement achieved by Nialamide was more prominent in regard to alertness and degree of communication while the patients did reveal very little change regarding action, emotion and intellection. The two patients who got worse showed increased hostility.

Although the results of this experiment with Nialamide for listless and apathetic geriatric patients are modest only, it is my feeling that they were encouraging and worthy of consideration and further study.

IV. Psychopharmacological Drugs for Confused Geriatric Patients

The confused geriatric patient represents a great problem in psychiatric hospitals. A great number of geriatric patients are hospitalized because they become disoriented, show impairment of their memory (especially for recent events), get confused, wander around, find themselves "lost" and eventually are picked up on the streets by helpful police or sometimes by irritated neighbors. Frequently they are unable to find their way back home by themselves and occasionally become victims of car or train accidents. Although a slight to moderate degree of confusion might be due, according to my own observations, to emotional conflicts with a great amount of anxiety, the majority of my geriatric patients revealed signs of moderate or severe confusion as a symptom of an Acute or Chronic Brain Syndrome and were found urgently in need of hospitalization and treatment. Stimulated by publications of J. D. Smigel, L. N. Sarhus and S. Barmak (142), by N. Seidel, A. A. Silver, and N. Nagel (132), by S. Levy (103) who found the use of metrazol in tablet form useful for confused elderly patients, and by published improvements, especially in regard to attention span and memory, I had, in 1955, made a study using metrazol for geriatric patients.

Twenty-four elderly patients were treated with metrazol in combination with nicotinic acid for a period of six months. The initial dosage was 200 mg., twice daily. After one month the dose was doubled. The average age of these patients was 69 years. Thirty percent of these patients improved considerably after a period of four months. They became more sociable, more alert, better oriented, showed improvement of memory for recent events, and became more interested in activities. One patient became nauseated, another got convulsions which ceased when metrazol was discontinued. The majority of these patients were diagnosed as Chronic Brain Syndrome associated with Cerebral Arteriosclerosis, with psychotic reaction.

Furthermore, two very interesting studies have been made with the use of Glutamic Acid (Monosodium L'Glutamate) combined with multi-vitamins in form of L'Glutavite. The first was effected with cooperation of H. E. Himwich, A. L. Hunsicker, and W. A. Himwich (79) in 1954, at the Galesburg State Research Hospital (Ill.). The second was carried out at the Osawatomie State Hospital (Kansas). (159) In the experiment done at the Galesburg State Research Hospital, 27 geriatric patients took part. Of these 27, 17 were judged improved: 16 in regard to "action." These patients took more active part in occupational therapy and showed more interest in their work. Twelve patients became more optimistic and cheerful. Nine of these 27 patients showed improved intellectual functioning, increased power of calculation and better recall of recent events. Eight achieved happier interpersonal relationships. They became friendlier, more sociable, more communicative and revealed a better ward adjustment. Five of these patients showed a change in their thought processes, which became faster, and finally two revealed increased "insight," as their delusional systems became less compelling and were regarded more critically. The average age of the patients was 65. The average dosage was 10 grams, three times daily. This dosage was given for a period of three months; then for a period of four weeks, placebo was used; and finally Monosodium L'Glutamate was started again for three more months. Frequent clinical observations and psychological testing before, during and after the medication were made. Biological studies measuring the level of glutamic acid in the blood did not reveal an increase of that substance in the blood. It could not be proved that glutamic acid was able to penetrate the blood-brain barrier and enter the brain. However, an adrenergic action of glutamic acid and rise of glucose in the blood appeared to be cause for the action of glutamic acid on the emotional status. Side effects were not observed in this study. One patient died very suddenly of coronary thrombosis during the experiment.

In the second experiment using Monosodium L'Glutamate, combined with multi-vitamins, 30 geriatric patients suffering predominantly from Chronic Brain Syndrome associated with Cerebral Arteriosclerosis or Senility were involved in a double-blind study.

The average age of the patients was 69 years. The first group of 15 patients was treated with glutamic acid for three months, after which they were put on placebo for one more month. The second group of 15 patients was given the placebo for an initial period of three months, glutamic acid during the next three months and finally placebo again for one month. Of the 30 patients in this study, 20 showed good to fair improvement, which centered upon such factors as alertness, orientation, interpersonal relationships and interest in occupational and recreational activities. Confusion and verbal incoherence was decreased, while on the other hand no significant effect on memory had been observed. Side effects were mild: Two patients became hyperactive; one suffered from an allergic dermatitis which improved after decrease of the dosage. The dose used for this experiment was 3.5 gm. Monosodium L'Glutamate, three times daily before meals, in tomato juice.

These favorable results achieved by the use of Monosodium L'Glutamate for confused geriatric patients have been confirmed recently in experiments done by R. D. Currier, M. E. Smith, E. H. Steinberger, and M. Steininger (42). In another study, done by M. Gasster (62), geriatric patients revealed improvement in regard to memory defects because of the application of Monosodium L'Glutamate. This author found the results obtained with Monosodium L'Glutamate to be superior to the ones obtained with metrazol.

For a number of years, special research has been done at the Parhon Institute of Geriatrics, in Bucharest, Roumania, in regard to treatment of the aging process. Anna Aslan (5, 6), after intensive experimental studies on animals, has treated more than 1400 patients in the older age group with procaine hydrochloride, 2%, in form of injections. Aslan has noted, also, improvement in memory, attention, interest and activity in geriatric patients.

In an experiment at the VA Hospital, Coatesville (Pa.), the results obtained by Aslan in regard to improvement of memory and confusion could not be confirmed. (162) In cooperation with J. Klugler, 14 male geriatric patients were given procaine injections, 2%. Their average age was 64 and their mean length of hospitalization 14 years. They were given injections three times weekly for four weeks and then, after an interval of 10 days, the treatment was repeated. Physical and psychiatric evaluation was given before, in between, and after the experiment. Laboratory tests included urine examination, blood count, and EKG. No side effects had been observed. The results of the experiment, however, were disappointing. Three patients became more alert. One of these also became more cheerful and the other one more active and cooperative. A fourth patient felt physically stronger and less fatigued and showed a better appetite and consequently increased a few pounds of weight. None of these 14 patients revealed any improvement in regard to orientation, memory or confusion.

In regard to treatment of confusion in the geriatric patient, we have to take into account the fact that a moderate degree of confusion is not always due to brain damage but can be caused by emotional factors exclusively. A confused state in the elderly patient, with feelings of being lost and bewildered, without permanent impairment of orientation or memory, could be a reaction to loss of a beloved object or to changes in the environment, such as in employment or in social status. Elderly persons resent such changes and might also become deeply concerned and confused after retirement from an occupation which has been their goal and purpose in life, or even during a physical sickness such as increasing difficulty in hearing or decreased eyesight, which frequently plagues them. In such cases, psychotherapy is indicated and of value.

D. MILIEUTHERAPY

I. Occupational Therapy.
II. Recreational Activities.

III. Music Therapy.
IV. Industrial Therapy.
V. Educational Therapy.
VI. Physical Therapy and Hydrotherapy.
VII. Habit Training.

I. Occupational Therapy with the Geriatric Patient

The importance of an active occupational therapy program for the chronically ill and the aged has been described by A. B. C. Knudson (94), M. B. Ferderber (55), H. Blustein (15) and others. The Veterans Administration has recognized the value of occupational therapy for the rehabilitation of the geriatric patient and is now striving to improve occupational therapy activities in a progressive rehabilitation service in its hospitals throughout the country. Important research has been done at the Veterans Administration Hospital in Downey, Illinois, and the good results of the new approach in regard to the treatment of geriatric patients have been described by Blustein. Blustein recommends a special occupational therapy program for elderly veterans using many varieties of handiwork with simple tools and devices. These include leather work, wood-working, basketry, weaving, painting, knotting, hooking rugs, knitting, and copper tooling. Their attention span was limited to 45 minutes. Library clubs were started by librarians for the purpose of giving book reviews and discussing current events. The patients helped in special assignments on the wards: making beds, helping others to make beds, arranging linen in the linen room, mending clothing, dusting areas around their bed. Hobbies were encouraged, like keeping scrapbooks, making joke books, cutting out cartoons and pasting them in books. An aquarium was maintained on the ward and interest in nature study was encouraged.

According to my own experience with occupational therapy with geriatric patients in psychiatric institutions, I have found an active occupational program of great usefulness, and I strongly recommend it.

Occupational therapy for geriatric patients in mental institutions and clinics has been prescribed for many years, but usually only for its physical or orthopedic benefits. This kind of occupational therapy was directed toward the maintenance of bodily function in patients with rheumatoid arthritis or hemiplegia, toward the rehabilitation of patients with fractures, and toward improving circulation, the function of muscles and joints, and coordination in neurological diseases.

Today, occupational therapy is employed more for its benefit in alleviating psychological and sociological problems. G. S. Fidler (57) and J. W. Fidler believe that occupational therapy is "a set form of psychiatric treatment which uses constructive activity as a modus operandi." W. C. Menninger (117) recommends hobbies, recreational and occupational therapy to release tension, to compensate for real or fancied inadequacies, to decrease feelings of inferiority and to give outlets for restlessness and hostility.

Generally, I prefer having elderly male and female patients working in a group together. This makes it possible to form attachments by visiting each other while working on their projects. It also tends to improve their personal habits. Sometimes such a close relationship leads to a marriage of an elderly couple after the end of the hospitalization and enhances motivations for leaving the hospital. The couples who do occupational therapy work together usually take a greater interest in recreational and outdoor activities, too, and the relationship between them helps their adjustment at the hospital remarkably.

Studying the application of occupational therapy for geriatric patients for many years has helped me to make the following observations: The preferred occupational therapy for men is woodwork consisting of making waste baskets, doll furniture, magazine tables or end tables. The men also like to do weaving, link belts, rake knitting and plastic lace work; while the women prefer mending, crocheting, embroidery, piecing quilts, making doll clothes and sewing carpet strips. Both men and women enjoy gardening. The men do the heavy digging and clean the space for flowers; the women plant the seeds and take care of the ground; both are happy going out on the ground and picking a bouquet.

The goal with occupational therapy in the geriatric group is essentially the same as with any other group of patients: Elderly individuals need to gain self-esteem, become more self-confident, develop friendships and learn to express their aggressive drives in a socially acceptable and more controlled manner.

For increasing their self-esteem at the beginning of the treatment, simple projects should be started. Crafts used for this purpose may include waffle-weave mats, jersey loop potholders, wood burning and simple, easily completed wood projects such as doorstops, tie racks, and small footstools. As soon as the geriatric patients are ready to try more difficult projects, the women may begin braid weaving on the upright loom or crocheting or making doll clothes. The men go on to more advanced woodworking which includes doll furniture, small tables, sawing, wastepaper baskets, fence pickets, or a combination of these projects.

To improve social life, the men, for instance, were requested to make doll beds while the women prepared doll mattresses, sheets, pillowcases. Soon the patients started to discuss their projects together.

For a better outlet of aggressivity, clay work was used, and sawing wood, nailing the parts together, and some sanding were recommended. Tearing of rags appeared to be useful, too.

In the geriatric group, a special effort has to be made to improve the patient's memory and concentration. To increase their faculty to remember, it has been found useful to let the patients do simple, repetitive projects which require the same step over and over. To teach concentration, the project has to be one requiring full attention.

It is infrequent that geriatric patients get disturbed during occupational therapy sessions. Generally they feel more satisfied, more needed and better accepted. I found it of value to have short sessions only, of no longer duration than one hour. Patients who have short attention spans should be encouraged to continue for a little longer than they may wish. The age of the patient, I observed, is not so great a handicap as the degree of physical disability.

It is, furthermore, of great importance that occupational therapy for geriatric patients should not consist of too minute or fine work. When planning projects for elderly patients, the individual eyesight, physical handicaps, and intelligence have to be taken into consideration. Geriatric patients usually need praise and encouragement.

A lasting and remarkable success for geriatric patients through occupational therapy is not easy to achieve. For the chronically ill patients it takes a longer period of time to respond to treatment because they have lost interest in their surroundings and often feel sorry for themselves. Acutely ill patients respond quicker to treatment once they can be induced to start it, because their interest has not been interrupted for very long. They are usually more active and want to participate in a group.

The following case history might be helpful to illustrate how a confused, disoriented and hostile geriatric patient can be helped by skillful application of occupational therapy.

CASE HISTORY

A 79 year old patient was admitted to a psychiatric hospital. The reason for his admittance was that he wandered away from his home in daytime, got lost on the streets, and could not find his way back. He talked incoherently and became confused, was completely out of contact, was disoriented in all three spheres, and became agitated at times. When placed in a nursing home, he was aggressive toward other inmates in the home, suffered from temper tantrums and, in fits of rage, destroyed furniture, tore bed sheets and his own clothing. He was brought to jail where he was put in restraint because of his destructive tendencies, and from jail he was finally transferred to the hospital for treatment.

At the hospital he was put on Thorazine medication for a number of weeks and became quieter. His temper tantrums subsided in a couple of days and he was taken out of seclusion. Still completely out of contact, he talked in a rambling, confused and threatening manner to the aides and was taken out of his room to join an occupational therapy group of about 20 males and 20 females. At the beginning he refused to do any kind of work, threw wooden projects of other patients on the floor and ran away from the occupational therapy room.

I approached him daily, talked to him in very simple words about the occupational therapy tools and what could be done with them, encouraging him to try them. Again he refused and talked in a threatening way. He was spoken to for about 10 days. Then one day he watched, with some interest, the work which one of the female patients was doing, and said that she reminded him of his sister. The occupational therapy worker became attentive and let both of these patients sit together. After two more days, the patient volunteered to help to put some nails into a doll bed. The two patients finally started to get better acquainted. The next day, the patient wanted to help paint the doll bed. He was unable to handle the brushes, however. The occupational therapy worker helped him to do so in a friendly, encouraging way. When he finished the painting, the psychiatrist came and praised his work. The next day the patient smiled for the first time and, while continuing with his painting job, said some coherent words to the other patients and to the occupational therapist. The following day he asked to do a doll bed by himself, cutting the wood with a saw and putting the pieces together. The occupational therapist, anxious about giving the patient a saw and concerned about what he might do with it, asked the psychiatrist for advice. I agreed to the patient's wish but together with the occupational therapist I watched carefully how the patient handled the tools. The patient did a perfect job and became more and more confident and talkative. He talked less confusedly, was friendlier, and asked for more difficult jobs. He was put on a wooden sled project, building the sled and painting it, again, together with the female patient. He did an excellent job and was praised for it.

After six months this patient became oriented to time and place, talked coherently and was in good contact. He was friendly and cooperative, took part in all activities on the ward, liked to dance with "his sister" and showed much enjoyment in folk dances. He participated in bingo games and offered a sled as a gift to the psychiatrist, with whom he talked about his interest in farming and carpenter work. He considered doing carpentry work at home to earn some money so that he could feel that "my family will be proud of me and will not consider me useless and too old to do anything." Then he stated that "if my wife does not know how many things I can do, I will take my sister home with me, and we will have a good time together."

This patient, who seemed to be, on arrival at the hospital, a "hopeless" case, was released from hospitalization after eight months.

II. Recreational Activities

No activity has been less understood and more abused than recreation. For many people recreational activities mean merely entertainment from which the patients get some enjoyment, like dancing, going to movies, watching television, hearing music on records, or watching sports. For elderly persons, the proper approach to these activities is thought by some to be a more passive one because elderly individuals are believed to be physically unable or not mentally alert enough for active participation in recreational activities.

This approach appears to me to be ineffective. First of all, recreation never means entertainment, but a return to a creative life, a salvage of something that has been lost or is in danger of being lost. It means, according to M. Gumpert (75), restoration of, or the growth of, functions which have been abused or neglected in the routine of living. While work is a state of tension and leisure is characterized by a release from work-tension, meaningful relaxation is the necessary consequence of, and is conducive to, a new rhythmic flow of life which precedes, leads to, and inspires creative work. If we lived in continuous tension—as many rigid and compulsive personalities do, without giving themselves time to relax, to experience leisure, to repose—the natural rhythm of life would be severely disturbed. No human being can remain physically and emotionally healthy by living in continuous tension but is in need of a recharge of his energies which restores the creative force in us. Life without relaxation would be monotonous and is a sign of becoming inflexible and more and more mechanical. Work done in this dull milieu is almost certain to be unimaginative and unoriginal. Humanity needs both work and relaxation to feel complete, just as it must experience the state of being awake and being asleep, day and night, stormy and calm waters of the ocean, like moonlight and sunshine, birth and death. We may call it the rhythm of life.

When we disturb artificially this rhythm, we destroy nature around us and natural feelings in us.

To keep, to maintain, to restore the normal rhythm of life, compulsive human beings are in need of recreation. Therefore, recreational activities have a meaning, a purpose, a goal of great importance. For elderly persons, recreational activities are necessary and of value when they create an atmosphere of release from tension, of relaxation and when they "charge" them with new energy. Recreation can give a new direction to an older person's life and help him to find and to develop possibilities of emotional growth and intellectual understanding which the elderly individual has not dreamed of.

Recreational activities, therefore, are a means toward a well-defined goal. They should not be seen as technical procedures only but should be used individually and with skill to develop and maintain a new creative life. For this reason, it becomes necessary to understand the geriatric patients, to have a good knowledge of their assets, and to learn about their hidden or forgotten talents and faculties, their unfulfilled wishes and intellectual desires, their motivation and their dreams. Like "Grandma" Moses, an elderly individual might be able to discover talents after the age of 70 and start a new, more complete, more happy and harmonious life.

According to A. Reid Martin (110), we are dealing in our everyday life mainly with what could be called "compulsive living" rather than "leisurely living." Compulsive intellectual preoccupation with one's internal problems is a characteristic symptom of many of our patients, young or old. "Creative insight," E. D. Hutchinson (81) pointed out, never occurred during the peak of mental effort, but always during a period of relaxation. Relaxation, decrease of tension, and leisure are needed and achieved by recreational techniques which help us to return to a new, more creative life. Such recreational activities can be undertaken by watching a movie or television, by sport activity (hunting, fishing, and others), hobbies (like stamp collecting), by reading books or magazines, gardening, planting flowers, caring for animals, sculpturing, working with clay, embroidery work, sewing, cooking, by wandering and observing nature (birds, animals, minerals) and many other activities. The recreational techniques to be used, with the purpose of relaxing the elderly patient, have to be chosen with great care and understanding of the elderly individual's assets, previous interests and limitations. These limitations can be as much of physical as of intellectual or emotional nature and should be evaluated by a competent recreational worker, with the help of a psychiatrist, before therapy is started. It is evident that very active athletic activities wherein the individual is forced and encouraged to compete with others are less suitable for most geriatric patients and might only induce to greater tension and ruin our therapeutic goal. More passive activities might be indicated at times for the purpose of relaxaation. Many elderly individuals, however, possess unknown qualities not discovered or not sufficiently used. Making it possible for them to use their assets and possibilities more purposefully and efficiently might help them to improve their emotional and physical health and restore them to many years of happy and creative life. According to W. Menninger (117), the elderly person with a hobby is almost always an alert, interesting person. Recreation is an extremely important aid to growing older gracefully. People who stay young despite their years do so because of an active interest that provides satisfaction through participation.

III. Music Therapy

Music therapy for the geriatric patient appears to me a still-neglected but promising field which definitely has a place in his psychiatric treatment. I have found rhythm bands useful in awakening their interest in communications and socialization. Many geriatric patients found enjoyment in rhythm bands, started to participate with encouragement and sometimes showed a happy smile for the first time after many years. Music is an excellent means of arousing their interest and furthering their craving to belong. For example, playing a drum in an orchestra can help them to express and sublimate some of their hostility. Singing in a choir can stimulate their interest in religious participation and in other group activities. Finally, folk dances, for male and female patients in better contact with their environment already, might help them to get not only better adjusted in the hospital but also to take interest in other persons and is of definite value to geriatric patients prior to their release from hospitalization when they return to community life or are placed in foster or old-age homes where they meet persons of their own age and of the opposite sex. According to my experience, talking to members of the other sex, eating together with them in a dining room, and having recreational activities or dances with them, is a great necessity for geriatric patients who lived in a hospital environment for many years and have forgotten how to behave with members of the opposite sex in public.

IV. Industrial Therapy

Industrial assignments have proved to be worth while for geriatric patients who need a goal and purpose in life and acceptance by the younger generation. Elderly patients, unless physically sick, can do many more things than we generally expect. With sufficient support they can often become conscientious clerks, gardeners, messengers or cooks in a psychiatric hospital and may often do well in a member-employee program. Sometimes they work with greater diligence and patience than younger patients.

V. Educational Therapy

Educational therapy may be of value after careful consideration of the geriatric patient's assets and limitations. The discovery and utilization of hobbies and interests, for instance reading books or magazines, learning a foreign language, participation in classes for accounting or typing, can be of value in the management of geriatric patients. One 64 year old male, who was uncommunicative, listless and uninterested for more than 12 years of his hospitalization, during one of my psychiatric interviews revealed interest in poetry and read to me a few poems he had written during the last year and kept carefully hidden in his pockets. He was praised and encouraged to write more poems, which were published in the hospital's patients' newspaper. From this time on the patient's emotional condition started to improve, slowly but constantly; he began to talk to other patients, became more interested in ward activities, lost his seclusive and shy attitude completely, and was considered for a release from hospitalization after seven months. The history of this patient is only one of very many known to me in which, by the intensive interest of the psychiatrist in, and an adequate utilization of a patient's assets, his mental condition improved considerably.

VI. Physical Therapy and Hydrotherapy

Physical therapy and hydrotherapy have also been found of value for geriatric patients. According to Blustein, (15) at the Veterans Administration Hospital, Downey, Illinois, electrical stimulation combined with Buerger-Allen exercises for circulatory disturbances in the lower extremities, general conditioning exercises using the stationary bicycle, individual exercises—especially posture exercises to prevent complications of inactivity—were used with success. According to my own experience, cold baths, scotch douches and active exercises, friction with cold water and general massage were frequently effective against symptoms of general weakness, fatigue and tiredness for elderly patients. However, all these techniques and exerciss should be used only with caution and under constant supervision. Too much exercise and too-frequent hydrotherapeutic applications might be of damage to the geriatric patient. We should be aware of the fact that although we can use these techniques against the symptoms of fatigue successfully in some geriatric patients, they are no substitute for psychiatric treatment of the feelings of weakness and exhaustion which can be eliminated only when we are able to recognize the emotional factors involved and treat them accordingly.

VII. Habit Training

Another factor of great concern is the geriatric patient's toilet habits. The more regressed a patient gets, the worse his personal hygiene becomes. He might soil his clothing, not be able to control his urine or bowel function, show food particles on his shirt, burn his pants with cigarettes, remain unkempt, unshaved, and wash only when supervised. This deterioration of the geriatric patient's toilet habits gets more frequent with increasing age and represents one of the symptoms of senility. To combat deterioration of toilet habits in elderly patients, a strict routine of washing, cleaning, changing beds, bathing the patients at regular hours, and a strict bedpan routine or the method of bringing the patients to the toilet at two-hour intervals in daytime and three-hour intervals at nighttime has been proved successful, in some cases. However, according to my own experience, bedwetting of elderly patients represents, at times, not only a physical symptom of bladder weakness or paralysis but is used by the patient to express his anger, resentment and hostility because of his feelings of being neglected and not getting enough attention or loving care.

I believe that toilet training, too, has to be done by psychological means. When a geriatric patient feels secure and protected, when his feelings of resentment decrease, when he discontinues considering his ward nurse as an authoritative mother figure punishing him for his faulty habits and "pushing him around," or, when he gets on friendly terms with the nursing personnel, the patient's toilet training improves remarkably. Therefore, a rigid, authoritative routine cannot become a substitute for understanding, patience and loving attention. This appears to be the mistake of many toilet training methods. An adequate training of the nursing personnel, which have to participate in the psychiatric program of rehabilitation of the geriatric patient, appears to be the only way of improving faulty toilet habits of the elderly when caused by emotional factors.

It is a fact that the successful therapy of the geriatric patient in a psychiatric institution should combine all these different methods and techniques of milieu therapy. Collaboration of the occupational therapy, recreational therapy, and physical therapy departments is necessary. Only a combined, active and comprehensive program under the direction of a physician who knows the physical handicaps of his patients and the emotional factors involved in his patients' sickness, can result in therapeutic success and, consequently, in rehabilitation.

6

POST-HOSPITALIZATION CARE

I. The Day (or Night) Hospital System.
II. Nursing Home Care.
III. Day Care Centers.
IV. Half-Way Houses and Community Activities.

I. THE DAY (OR NIGHT) HOSPITAL SYSTEM

It is general policy that no geriatric patient, once in remission from his psychosis or recovered from his confusion or disturbed behavior, should be permitted to leave the psychiatric institution without a plan for continuous treatment outside the hospital. If he has sufficient economic means, the best treatment is by his own family physician who has known the patient for many years prior to referring him to the psychiatric hospital. A letter of special recommendations, with a copy of the patient's psychiatric case record, should be in the private physician's hands before the patient returns to his home environment. The hospital psychiatrist has to explain the patient's psychodynamics and make understandable to the family doctor why and how the geriatric patient got disturbed, confused or psychotic, what kind of stress situation possibly caused his hospitalization and the patient's underlying personality structure. Furthermore, not only a diagnosis should be given but also a prognostic indication in regard to the possibility of future relapses of the patient, causing his eventual return to the hospital. Such a private and personal communication to the family physician should indicate, too, what medication (for instance, tranquilizers or energizers) have been given in the hospital with the exact dosage and, if possible, a recommendation by the psychiatrist that he wants the patient to continue his medication. The family physician should also be informed as to what other kind of psychiatric treatment has been given in the hospital—electrical shock treatment, for instance, individual or group psychotherapy, occupational, educational or recreational therapy, and others—so that the private physician might be able to continue with this treatment or change it as necessity arises according to his judgment and his own observations.

The greatest danger of a relapse of the geriatric patient's emotional trouble is never greater than when a treatment is discontinued completely once the patient is released from hospitalization and then left to his own devices. At times the elderly patient returns to the same situation of stress or strain involving rejection by other members of his family, by his own children, by his spouse. They might not have been informed about the psychological causes of the patient's abnormal behavior and go on treating him in a domineering way, belittling his efforts to remain active and creative or to find an adequate outlet in recreational activities or hobbies. They repeat the mistake of taking responsibilities from the elderly person which he is able to handle, and further his regression due to lack of understanding. Therefore, a thorough explanation of the patient's emotional condition to his family physician and, through him, to other members of the patient's family, is necessary and indicated. Without this advice, the patient's return to hospitalization can be expected sooner or later. With adequate treatment at home, however, the geriatric patient's relapse into his emotional sickness can be avoided frequently.

In psychiatry, as in general medicine, the medical world gets more and more aware of the fact that the patient's sickness should not be treated simply by treating the individual alone. All members of the family play an important role and, consciously or unconsciously, are a factor to be considered in regard to the origin, the recovery or the relapse of an individual's emotional sickness. Therefore, our goal in geriatric psychiatry today is adequate treatment of the whole family or "the family constellation." This might involve interviews with the members of the family in the presence of the patient or without the patient being present. I believe that almost always our success or failure in psychiatric therapy depends upon our advice, recommendations or treatments given to the sick individual's relatives. We will have to understand that the disturbed interpersonal relationships are not the problem of the patient alone, and that the patient is only part of his family. The family as a whole must be treated as it is recommended by N. W. Ackerman (2). According to Ackerman, the individual is only a mirror image, a microcosm of his family group. The diagnosis of emotional illness and health cannot be restricted to the individual; it must encompass the individual within the group and the group as well. The ills of individuals, families, and society are interrelated.

In case the patient has no family physician of his own or no means to afford a private doctor, the hospital psychiatrist still remains responsible for the patient's continuous observation and treatment after his release from the hospital. Adequate therapeutic methods have to be made continuously available in order to prevent relapses into the emotional sickness of the elderly patient.

There are many possibilities open to the psychiatrist from which to choose, according to the patient's mental condition and emotional needs. They are the day (or night) hospital system, the outpatient departments or mental hygiene clinics, the halfway houses, and the nursing homes. Of growing importance, too, are recreational day centers like the Sirovich Day Center or the Hodson Day Center in New York City or the Senior Citizen Center in San Francisco, which I consider to be of definite value for the maintenance of good emotional health among our Senior Citizens.

The idea of the day (or night) hospital is not a new one. Perhaps the oldest of this kind is at Gheel in Belgium. Well-known also is the day hospital at the Allan Memorial Institute in Montreal, Canada, under the direction of D. E. Cameron, and the day hospital of the Menninger Foundation in Topeka, Kansas. At the present time, many state and VA hospitals in the United States are using the day hospital system. In Europe, day hospitals have been emphasized, especially in Great Britain. While day hospitals in the United States have been built more for the purpose of post-hospitalization care, in England many patients receive their initial treatment in day hospitals and are not necessarily hospitalized in full-time hospitals. At the Marlborough Day Hospital, modern psychopharmacological drugs and occupational activities are the treatment of choice, while at the Travistock Clinic, near London, individual psychotherapy is given extensively.

In England, the Cowley Road Hospital, which, under the direction of L. Z. Cosin, is using the day hospital program with great success for geriatric patients, has become of great importance. To this day hospital report patients not in need of hospitalization who are treated with occupational therapy, physical therapy and an active retraining in the technique of social and daily living while living in their own homes. The emphasis is to avoid chronic hospitalization of geriatric patients. This new system has shown remarkable results.

According to Cosin (38, 39), a geriatric patient disturbed or confused, or suffering from physical sickness of a more serious kind will be admitted immediately to the geriatric unit. Cosin thinks it is recommendable to treat the vicious circle of family anxiety stress increasing anxiety, depression and dementia in the old person. For patients unable to pay their own family doctor, the geriatric unit's social worker and doctor are responsible for his follow-up outside the hospital. Cosin also recommends intermittent readmission for summer holidays and at other times during the year when stress on the family group begins to increase, when the situation has been observed by the social worker. The geriatric patient is readmitted immediately to the geriatric unit in the event of serious illness affecting the elderly patient or other members of the family group. Cosin emphasizes maintenance of optimal emotional and physical health for the geriatric patient by utilizing physical medicine and occupational therapy with a very active approach, while group psychotherapy is used, at the Oxford Unit, only to a minor degree. All geriatric patients with emotional disturbances are treated, however, by a psychiatrist.

According to Cosin, about 25% of 1000 patients admitted yearly suffer from severe mental disturbance, and 11%, or about 100 a year, have had long-standing emotional disturbances. About 38% of these 100 patients are eventually discharged to their homes; 7% are resettled in private nursing homes or long-stay annexes. Seventeen percent die of intercurrent infection, 9% are "certified" and transferred to mental hospitals. Only 19% generally remain residents at the Oxford Unit four to 10 months after admission. Three-quarters of the discharged patients attend the day hospital from one to five days a week and are helped to stay outside the hospital by this means. Very few of the day hospital patients need emergency readmission. The average age of the patients treated at the Oxford Day Hospital is 78 years.

Many hospitals in the United States now are using the system of day hospitals but some of them also include the night hospital method which permits patients to get treatment after working hours. They are permitted to sleep in the hospital and receive treatment more suitable for them when already employed but still in need of support.

There is no doubt that the idea of the day and night hospital has great promises for the future, especially for patients in the older age group, and needs to be developed further.

As W. Polner (124) has pointed out, the advantages of the day hospital for geriatric patients is not only of economic nature because the total cost per day is considerably less than the cost of hospitalization in an inpatient facility but also the greatest advantage lies in the fact that the patient keeps his place in the family and support is given not only to the patient but also to other members of the patient's family, relieving them from many anxieties and making it possible for them to work during the time the patient is at the day hospital. However, according to Polner, possible disadvantages in the day hospital program might result from the fact that the home environment is not always the most suitable for the patient and might undo some of the therapeutic work done with and for the patient at the hospital. Another aged person might also impose great strain on other members of the family at home. In the United States, in contrast to Great Britain, Canada, and some European countries, the day hospital program is recommended for indigent patients only, while the private physician's responsibilities are stressed. It is felt here that more benefit can be derived in training the general practitioner himself to treat more effectively his geriatric patients after hospitalization. However, in cases where day hospital treatment is economically and psychologically indicated, the intensive and competent treatment of the day and night hospital program with a minimum disruption of family life and community living is a necessity and of great importance for our geriatric patient population.

At the present, many large cities have such day hospitals in the United States as well as in Western Europe. They are in close affiliation with clinics and hospitals. During the last couple of years, the idea of the day hospital and its usefulness has grown and many day hospitals have been built in connection with state mental hospitals and Veterans Administration Hospitals, where young and older patients are observed and treated, under the supervision of psychiatrists or a psychiatric team which might include also a psychologist, a social worker, and an occupational therapist or recreation specialist. Also, in some of these day hospitals, geriatric patients, released from hospitalization, are treated by individual and group psychotherapy and take part in many occupational or recreational activities. In this way, the geriatric patient (as are children, young adults and middle-aged persons of both sexes) is treated according to his needs, and therefore relapses into a psychotic condition are frequently prevented.

II. NURSING HOME CARE

In 1959, about 4 to 6% of elderly individuals over 65 lived in various institutions; about 33,000 in homes for the aged, 450,000 in nursing homes, 141,000 in mental hospitals, and 26,000 in other hospitals. Approximately half of these nursing homes are proprietary, while the others belong to state or federal governments, church organizations or other private charity organizations. It is evident that the number of aged persons over 65 in nursing homes is increasing in proportion to a general increase of the aging population. Although many states have enforced rigid standards for nursing home care and supervision which requires medical treatment, adequate nursing care and equipment, including standards for bed space, fire prevention, bathing facilities, kitchen hygiene and others, there are still, unfortunately, "old age homes" or "boarding homes" which are not at the level of the licensed nursing homes and should be eliminated. The duties and responsibilities of the nursing home administrator which are various and difficult have been outlined by J. Kaplan (88), director of the Mansfield Memorial Homes, Inc., in Ohio. These duties include: having a thorough knowledge and understanding of the basic concepts, philosophy, and current trends in gerontology; interpreting problems of the aged to special publics when requested; and utilizing the modern principles of public, social welfare, hospital, and business administration. Most important, however, in addition to providing for adequate shelter, hygienic methods, nursing care, medical treatment when it becomes necessary, individualized meals according to dietary and other requirements of the older generation, the nursing home administrator must be able to understand the emotional needs of his clients. He has to keep them in contact with the community aspect of life, furnish adequate recreational and occupational activities in the home, encourage all kinds of hobbies, fulfill the elderly person's religious interests, and keep a good balance between the elderly citizen's wanting to "disengage himself" at times from the outside world and remain in a desired state of "individual separation," and the same person's cravings, at other items, toward human contact, to socialize, to play games with others and to share activities.

Of great importance appears to be the elderly individual's attitude toward members of his own family, his children and grandchildren. Elderly persons do not want to be considered a burden by members of their own family belonging to the younger generation, and at times put on a mask of wanting to stay aloof and isolated. Frequently, however, behind their air of aloofness, the need to meet their own children and grandchildren is very great and they actually become alive and happy again in their company. At other times, when bothered by the physical ailments, so frequent in elderly people, they do want to be alone and do not wish their children or grandchildren to know about these matters. Not infrequently, elderly persons need relatively more time for sleep and rest; they tire more easily and show features of fatigue. Therefore, the time element of visits with the younger generation is for them of great importance. Visits of too long duration might be resented by elderly citizens. Elderly individuals also are much in need of "meditation." They like to think about problems which are different from the ones of the younger generation. They have other ideas about "life" and the many activities in which young people are interested. They might not be able to understand some of the cravings and ambitions of the younger generation in a changing world.

Therefore, a certain equilibrium between the elderly person's passive meditative attitude, conducive to disengagement and wanted isolation, and his wish to participate in the life of younger people and feel part of their group is, according to my own experience with elderly people, a very important factor in handling them and keeping them happy and satisfied in nursing homes as well as in psychiatric institutions. A nursing home administrator, aware of these problems and able to handle them with tact and diplomacy, will surely contribute a great deal to the adjustment in the home and to the upholding of his clients' emotional equilibrium, his mental as well as physical health.

Whenever the elderly person gets emotionally disturbed or greatly confused or suffers from a physical sickness of a serious degree, transfer to a psychiatric institution or a general hospital might become a necessity. Therefore, no nursing home should be permitted to function without a psychiatric consultation service and adequate medical supervision, for the benefit and protection of the nursing home administrator as well as for the elderly clients.

I am very much in agreement with M. Leeds (100) who emphasizes that we find ourselves in a period of evolution of the home for the aged. The administrators of homes for the aged should act as an educational force and build close relationships with other medical facilities. The future home for the aged will be a complex geriatric facility that combines both medical care and fulfills the elderly citizen's needs for social, religious, recreational and occupational activities.

For this reason, in 1957, under my direction, in a state hospital in Kansas, special training courses were given for nursing home administrators, of four days' duration. They visited the state hospital and took part in lectures and seminars about geriatric psychiatry and observed, on the geriatric wards, the modern psychiatric treatment methods for elderly patients. In this way, the nursing home administrators not only bettered their knowledge and skill but the relationships between the psychiatric hospital and the nursing homes were improved. Furthermore, through better communication, the continuation of the geriatric patient's treatment after release from the hospital and transfer to a nursing home was furthered. Such a program is of definite value and should be introduced in all psychiatric institutions treating geriatric patients.

III. DAY CARE CENTERS

The treatment of the geriatric patient furthermore would be incomplete and unsatisfactory without the cooperation of a suitable day care center.

New York City has many excellently organized day care centers, sponsored by the Department of Welfare, the best known of which are the Hodson Center (founded 1943) and the Sirovich Day Center (opened 1949). They are usually open five days a week, admit elderly citizens of both sexes and without discrimination, have psychiatric and medical consultants and are under the direction of a trained social worker. In these centers the older person fills his unused day with activity that will stimulate and reactivate his hobbies, interests, assets and experiences and give him a feeling of accomplishment and usefulness. In these day centers the elderly persons work and play; they have their own hobby shops, do carpenter work, repair radios and television sets, build their own furniture, cook their own meals, mend their clothing, wash their laundry, paint pictures, study languages, learn or play musical instruments, singly or as an orchestra, meet in discussion groups, read books and magazines, have their own entertainment and even have their own poetry club where the elderly citizen reads and writes his own poetry. According to H. A. Levine (102), Consultant to and founder of the Hodson Center in New York City, activity for the older person is as essential to life as is food and shelter. Vegetating for the elderly is a form of deterioration and regression, leading to institutionalization and to slow death. A balanced program, taking into consideration his physical and emotional condition, can renew old interests and find new opportunities. In such a day center the elderly individual can meet people and make new friends and regain his feeling of belonging to a group. Group work programs are created and group activities are developed. Active participation and social activities are enhanced, and the elderly citizen learns again to carry responsibilities and gains new goals in life. Realistic attitudes toward life in general are assumed, and many new skills are learned, helping later in gainful employment, if so desired. These day centers, for elderly persons over 60, are valuable and useful institutions of our modern culture and are helpful in preventing emotional disturbances of the elderly by maintenance of their self-esteem and by letting them feel wanted, needed and accepted. When an elderly individual gets disturbed or confused, medical and psychiatric help is requested, preventing, frequently, hospitalization in a psychiatric institution.

There is no doubt that some of these day centers still suffer from lack of adequate personnel and equipment, but the idea of the day center is of value and should be developed further in the future.

According to S. Kubie and G. Landau (97), self-government is emphasized in day centers because the institution of self-government has proved to be one of the effective means of stimulating these older people to make use of their individual capacities. It has developed leadership, initiative, responsibility. It has also served to focus attention on, and increase identification with, the affairs of the center, even among the least participating members.

IV. HALF-WAY HOUSES AND COMMUNITY ACTIVITIES

Of growing importance for the rehabilitation of the geriatric patients not able to return to their own family is the utilization of other community resources. Such programs involve: placement in private families (foster homes); help with planning for suitable living arrangements in the community, residence hotels or apartment projects; meals-on-wheels; "friendly visitor" services by Red Cross or Volunteer groups; voluntary recreational facilities in the community such as Golden Age or Senior Citizens Clubs;

vocational guidance; placement in sheltered workshops; and legal guardianship advice. In England and in Australia, the "meals-on-wheels" service is emphasized because the philosophy behind such a service is that, frequently, elderly persons are not able to leave their own home due to physical sickness or emotional resistance and anxiety about meeting other people, or shame because of their condition. Furthermore, its value is enhanced by the fact that the "meals-on-wheels" program releases the elderly individual from the duties of preparing his own meal and permits him more time for recreational, occupational or other activities which would enhance his emotional and physical health. Such a service might also make it possible to release geriatric patients earlier from hospitalization. All these home services for elderly individuals should not take the initiative from the patient. They should not work against the geriatric patient's personal drive, ambition and motivation and should not make life too easy for him and, eventually, further his regression.

At home nursing, organized on a municipal or federal basis, may become a necessity for geriatric patients who are not in need of full-time nursing care and supervision in a nursing home and do not have financial means to provide these services on their own.

So-called "half-way houses" finally are becoming an increasing necessity. Such "half-way houses" represent a useful facility for geriatric patients who do not have a home or a family of their own, cannot be placed in a foster home, but are not in need of a psychiatric treatment program in a hospital or of continuous nursing care and supervision in a nursing home. The patients in this group work in the community during the day but return after their working hours to such a protective environment of a half-way house which is under the direction of a social worker, a nurse or a similarly experienced individual in the field of gerontology, able to give the elderly individual support when needed. Such a half-way house contains a greater number of patients than a foster home and has a closer communication system with the hospital from which the patients were released. This system of half-way houses, used extensively in England and gaining popularity in the United States, appears to me of usefulness for elderly patients not able yet to stand completely on their own feet and in need of support to find or hold a job, but definitely not requiring hospitalization any more.

The different types of programs concerned with the geriatric patient's emotional and physical health are many and vary according to the patient's needs. Therefore, skill, knowledge and flexibility are of greatest importance to the psychiatrist, who still shares the responsibility for the geriatric patient after his release from hospitalization. For this purpose, he has to utilize, on a highly individualized basis, not only the services of the patient's family physician but also the many services which the community has to offer. Therefore, a closer cooperation with the community and its organizations, which have to do things "with but not *for* the geriatric patients" is the proper approach to the solution of the continuously growing problem of our elderly individuals.

7

OUR GOAL: FROM CUSTODIAL CARE TOWARD REHABILITATION

In some psychiatric institutions we still find the elderly patient sitting with hopelessness and depression on his face, uninterested in his surroundings, listless, apathetic, and, at times, even neglected in his personal appearance—unkempt, unshaved, sloppy with his clothing, and more or less out of contact or mute. These patients convey the feeling of being outcasts of a society which does not care if they live or die, believing at times that "they would be better off dead" because "nothing can be done for them." They are "just old people waiting to die." The psychiatric ward of these patients looks depressing, too. There are no curtains, pictures or flowers, with the patients sitting near the walls, hardly talking to each other. Most of the time they are simply idle.

Fortunately, this "ward atmosphere" is slowly disappearing and is being replaced more and more by greater activity among the patients and an increasing interest by personnel in them. On many wards we find recreational activities such as card playing, Ping-pong, checkers, chess, television, radio music and occasional dances organized by volunteers or recreational workers. Nonetheless, the general attitude of the ward physician, nursing personnel, and the rest of the psychiatric team frequently remains one of hopelessness and depression and not being able to understand the whole situation or to do something about it.

What are the reasons? In regard to the psychiatrists, they frequently feel that elderly people are not approachable by psychotherapy because of their confusion, memory defects and delusional behavior. Others make an initial effort but find it difficult to have empathy with the elderly, lost patience and so then became discouraged because of their lack of success. Occasionally an elderly physician identifies with a geriatric patient but becomes depressed himself, especially if the elderly patient suffered from a heart condition or other physical ailment which the physician himself is afraid of developing, being of the same age. Other physicians get definitely hostile toward the geriatric patient because they are themselves deeply involved in an unresolved Oedipus complex. They may treat the female patients—if they themselves belong to the male sex—with great preference, sympathy and overindulgence, while the male geriatric patients are neglected or treated with too great strictness and control because they remind them of their own father. They become unconsciously vindictive and act out their resentment against their own father by unconsciously hating the patient. With the female physician, the roles may be reversed, but the underlying hostility sometimes comes into the open by threatening the patient with electric shock treatment or by taking their privileges away from them.

Therefore, it is of utmost importance, in the treatment of the geriatric patient, for the therapist to have an empathetic, understanding, supportive and loving attitude, together with objectivity and a mind open to understand the patient's problems. Also harmful is the tendency to slap the patient on the back, show pity and take away from him his responsibilities and his maturity. Elderly patients often act like children and overemphasize their helplessness in bathing, dressing or feeding. Nothing would be more incorrect than doing too much for them. It would only intensify their attitude of unresponsible helplessness, apathy and undignified dependency.

Another important problem to be kept in mind continuously when treating an elderly patient is the physician's and the patient's attitude toward old age generally and death particularly. Any person afraid of getting old and finding it depressing and fearful; any individual who is afraid to die and clings desperately to the delusion of his youthfulness will not be able to treat elderly patients successfully. A realistic philosophy toward life and death, based on the inevitability of growing old and dying and on the belief that death is part of living and basic to its fulfillment, is necessary in helping geriatric patients. Religion might be of assistance in overcoming the fear of dying. When a person's life has found full satisfaction—by creating a family or a piece of art, a contribution to science, or indeed by creating anything of use, enjoyment, of purposeful advancement for other people, a community or a country—death should not be a cause of fear but of meaningful rest, giving others a chance and a possibility to grow, to develop and to further one's own creation. When the psychiatrist is able to feel this way, and convey his calm and his hope by having overcome his own fear of death, when he himself has understood the full meaning of life, of growth and of sharing with others, when he is convinced that the younger generation has to develop its own creative efforts after careful consideration of what has been built by the older generation in the past, only then will the psychiatrist or the physician who treats the elderly have the possibility to understand them deeply and to show them the way out of emotional conflicts and worry, toward freedom, calm and serenity.

The goal of "successful aging," according to R. J. Havinghurst (76), should not be occasioned with only one particular life-style, whether it be one of activity or one of disengagement. Life satisfaction will probaby be associated with active involvement for some kinds of people. For others, disengagement will be the source of adjustment.

There is no simple theory of successful aging which can account for all the people in their later years. There is some disengaging force, to withdraw from society, in some persons over 70 or 80. But most of them will retain the attitude toward life of their middle years. Those who were happy and satisfied in their activity and productivity will then continue to be happy and satisfied if they can maintain a considerable part of their activity and productiveness. Those who were happy and satisfied by being relatively passive and dependent in their middle years, will be happy and satisfied if they can become even more disengaged in their later years.

Therefore, the problem of rehabilitation is not a simple one. It can be handled only on an individual basis. There are a few definite needs, however, which must be fulfilled if a human being is to remain emotionally healthy and not succumb to the many conflicts, abnormal reactions and moods accompanying the process of aging. The most outstanding needs, bringing unhappiness, dissatisfaction and emotional ill health, when not satisfied, are of physiological nature involving physiological body-growth, nourishment and organ function and of psychological nature, the need to feel safe from danger and threat, to belong to a group and to be loved, the need for prestige and recognition, for self-actualization and, for some persons, for aesthetic surroundings and for beauty.

The geriatric patient has lost many of his satisfactions; he considers himself "lost," without purpose, without goal, without direction. He is confused, believes himself frequently to be a burden and realizes, consciously or unconsciously, that life has no more meaning for him.

A rehabilitation program, therefore, should take into consideration the geriatric patient's present physical and mental condition in an objective and highly individualized way. It has to improve upon his physical condition and disabilities by means of all the scientific methods and treatments available to modern medicine, restoring, if possible, to the elderly patient's physical condition the physical strength and vigor of his former adult life, using physical therapy, hydrotherapy, drugs, diet, and corrective therapy when indicated. But such a rehabilitation program must give greatest importance to the emotional problem involved in order to restore a patient not only to his previous physical state of health but also to emotional equilibrium.

A. B. C. Knudson (94) advises that this type of health promotion would include rehabilitation techniques for the prevention of illness and disability, with the objective of halting impairment of health and onset of disability. The psychiatrist, with his rehabilitation team, should contribute a part of the total resources brought to bear in an aggressive approach in such a preventive program. Prior to any treatment program, a comprehensive health inventory should be made for each individual. Physical medicine and rehabilitation, according to Knudson, can be of real help in pre-vocational activities in determining and increasing work capacity, physical tolerance, mental alertness and emotional stability.

F. J. Braceland (18) is of the opinion that psychiatry and rehabilitation deal with two of the greatest adversities that befall mankind: mental and physical disaster, whether innate or acquired, acute or chronic, temporary or prolonged. They both work in the framework of the therapeutic environment and the therapeutic team and thus in the context of group dynamics. They deal with an individual who lives, feels, thinks, struggles, and expends his energy in defending himself against a threat to his integrity. Therefore, psychiatry and rehabilitation have to rehabilitate man *as man,* no matter how badly disabled he may be or how seriously restricted are his activities. The patient has to return to society a "complete person," skilled or perhaps newly-skilled in important techniques and especially in the art of living. A revision of his "body image" might become necessary, his conception of himself might have to be changed, and of his relations to others. For this purpose, the psychiatrist will have to work with the more mature aspects of the patient's personality in order to prevent chronic regression and lasting disability.

An adequate rehabilitation service of the geriatric patient therefore does include: restoring his physical health and preventing further physical disabilities by corrective and preventive treatment in an institution well-equipped for this purpose, and keeping the elderly patient in good emotional equilibrium by all means available to the psychiatrist or well-trained physician.

But such a rehabilitation service would still be of no avail, if given in the hospital environment only, without consideration of the patient's resocialization and rehabilitation in the circle of his family, his community, and his place of work and relaxation.

The goal and purpose of the rehabilitation program for the geriatric patient is, therefore, to restore and keep his physical strength and vigor, to help him regain his emotional equilibrium, disturbed by the factor of aging, and return him to the circle of his family and his community as a dignified and creative human being whose needs to be loved, accepted in and by a group, to feel needed and to have a high self-esteem, are satisfied. The aged patient has to become again part of humanity, adjusted as well as possible to the problems of a progressive world with faith in himself, in his future, and in others.

REFERENCES

1. Abraham, K.: The Applicability of Psychoanalytic Treatment to Patients at an Advanced Age. In *Selected Papers of Psychoanalysis.* London, Hogarth Press, 1949.
2. Ackerman, N. W.: *The Psychodynamics of Family Life.* Basic Books, Inc., 1958.
3. Alders, W.: The idea of a home for the aged: A reappraisal. *J. Am. Geriatrics Soc., IX*:11, 1961.
4. Alexander, F. G., and French, T. M.: *Psychoanalytic Therapy, Principles and Applications.* New York, Ronald Press, 1946.
5. Aslan, A.: A new method for the prophylaxis and treatment of aging with novocain. Eutropic and rejuvenating effects. *Therapiewoche,* 7:14-22, 1956.
6. Aslan, A.: Recent Experience on the Rejuvenating Action of Novocain (H3). In *Research on Novocain Therapy in Old Age.* New York, Consultants Bureau, Inc., 1959.
7. Ayd, F. J., Jr., A preliminary report on Marsilid. *A. J. Psychiat.,* 114, 459, 1957.
8. Barnard, R. I.; Robbins, L. L. and Tetzlaff, F. M.: *Day hospital* as extension of psychiatric treatment. *Bull. Menninger. Clin.,* 60, 1952.
9. Barnes, R. H.; Busse, E. W.; and Friedman, E. L.: The Psychological functioning of aged individuals with normal and abnormal electroencephalograms, II, A study of hospitalized individuals. *J. Nerv. & Ment. Dis., 124*:585-593, 1956.
10. Bellak, L.: *Schizophrenia.* A Review of the Syndrome. New York, Logos Press, 1958.
11. Benaim, S.: Group psychotherapy within a geriatric unit: An experiment. *Internat. J. Social Psychiat. III*:2, 1957.
12. Bettag, O. L.; Slight, D.; Wenig, P. W. and Sorensen, W. H.: The Aged and Aging in Illinois, Part I: The Mentally Ill. Springfield, Department of Public Welfare, 1955.

13. Birren, J. E.: Principles of Research on Aging. In: *Handbook of Aging and the Individual Psychological and Biological Aspects,* edited by J. E. Birren. University of Chicago Press, 1959.
14. Birren, J. E.: Sensation, Perception and Modification of Behavior in Relation to the Process of Aging, In Birren, J. E.; Imus, H. A. and Windle, W. F.: *The Process of Aging in the Nervous System.* Springfield, Thomas, 1959.
15. Blustein, H.: A rehabilitation program for geriatric patients. *J. Am. Geriatrics Soc., VII*: 3, 1960.
16. Bortz, E. L.: Healthy Added Years. *Encyclop. Britannica,* Inc., 1961.
17. Bortz, E. L.: Education, aging and meaningful survival. *J. Am. Geriatrics Soc., IX*:5, 1961.
18. Braceland, F. J.: The role of the psychiatrist in rehabilitation. *J.A.M.A.,* Sept. 21, 1957.
19. Bucke, M.: Leisure Time Activities of Elderly People in the United Kingdom. *The Gerontologist, I*:2, 1961.
20. Buerger, M.: *Altern und Krankheit, 3rd Edition.* Leipzig, Thieme, 1957.
21. Burgess, E. W.: Personal and Social Adjustment in Old Age. In *The Aged and Society,* Industrial Relations Research Association, edited by Milton Derber. Champaign, Twin City Printing Co., 1950.
22. Busse, E. W.; Barnes, R. H.; Silverman, A. J.; Thaler, M. and Frost, L. L.: Studies in the process of aging, X, the strengths and weaknesses of psychic functioning in the aged. *Am. J. Psychiat., 11*:896, 1955.
23. Busse, E. W.; Barnes, R. H.; Friedman, E. L. and Kelty, E. I.: Psychological functioning of aged individuals with normal and abnormal electroencephalograms. I. A study of non-hospitalized community volunteers. *J. Nerv. & Ment. Dis., 124*:135, 1956.
24. Busse, E. W.: Psychopathology. In *Handbook of Aging and the Individual,* edited by J. E. Birren. Univ. of Chicago Press, 1959.
25. Busse, E. W.: Problems affecting psychiatric care of the aging. *Geriatrics, 15*:10, 1960.
26. Butler, R. N.: Intensive psychotherapy for the hospitalized aged. *Geriatrics, 15*:9, 1960.

27. Caffey, E. M., Jr.; Hollister, L. E.; Pokorny, A. D.; and Bennett, L. J.: Tranquilizing and antidepressant drugs. *Med. Bulletin,* MB-6, Vet. Adm., Washington 25, D. C., Sept. 12, 1960.
28. Cameron, D. E.: The use of tofranil in the aged. *Canad. Psychiat. A. J., 4*:Supplement, 160-165, 1959.
29. Cameron, D. E.: The day hospital. *Modern Hospital,* 69, 1947.
30. Cameron, N.: Neuroses of Later Maturity. In O. J. Kaplan (Ed.), *Mental Disorders in Later Life, 2nd Edition.* Stanford, Cal., Univ. Press, 1956.
31. Casey, J. F.; Rackow, L. L. and Sperry, A. W.: Observations on the Treatment of the Mentally Ill in Europe. Vet. Adm., Washington 25, D. C., 1960.
32. Cashman, M. D.; and Lawes, T. G. G.: A controlled study of gerioptil. *British M. J.,* 554-556, Feb. 1961.
33. Chiu, G. C.: Rejuvenating effect of procaine. A critical review of reports. *J.A.M.A., 175*:6, 502-503, 1961.
34. Collins, G. B., and Mort, M.: Occupational therapy in a geriatric unit. *Brit. J. Phys. Med., 18*:9, 1955.
35. Coordinated Approach to Geriatrics. VA Regional Office, S. Francisco, Cal., 1953.
36. Cosin, L. Z.: The place of the day hospital in the geriatric unit. *Internat. J. Social Psychiat., 1*:33, 1955.
37. Cosin, L. Z.: Discussion on geriatric problems in psychiatry. *Proc. Roy. Soc. Med.,* Vol. 49, Nov. 8, 1955 (Section of Psychiatry).
38. Cosin, L. Z.: Geriatric day hospital for psychiatric patients. *M. World, 87*:214/219, 1957.
39. Cosin, L. Z.: Current Therapeutic and Psychotherapeutic Concepts for the Geriatric Patient. In *Progress in Psychotherapy,* edited by Masserman, J. H. and Moreno, J. L. New York, Grune and Stratton, 1957.
40. Crawshaw, R. S., and Peterson, L. K.: Supportive psychotherapy with an aged transient. *Geriatrics, 16*:9, 1961.
41. Cumming E.; Dean L. R.; Newell, D. S. and McCaffrey, J.: Disengagement—a tentative theory of aging. *Sociometry, 23*: 1, 1960.
42. Currier, R. D.; Smith, E. M.; Steininger, E. H. and Steininger, M.: A Study of L'Glutavite as compared to a ritalin combination in the chronic brain syndrome. *Geriatrics, 16*:6, 311-316, 1961.

43. Currier, M. E.; Helmle, M. and Caron, M.: Geriatric Habit Training. Report from the Pilgrim (N. Y.) State Hospital, 1952.

44. Dax, E. C.: The Accommodation and Treatment for Mentally Disturbed Geriatric Patients. In *Growing Old.* Problems of old age in the Australian Community, edited by Stoller, A. Melbourne, F. W. Cheshire, Publisher, First Edition, 1960.

45. Donahue, W.: Emerging Principles and Concepts. A Summary. In Donahue, W., and Tibbitts, C.: *The New Frontiers of Aging.* Ann Arbor, The Univ. of Michigan Press, 1957.

46. Donahue, W., and Tibbitts, C.: *Growing in the Older Years.* Ann Arbor, Univ. of Michigan Press, 1951.

47. Donavan, F.: Municipal Activities for the Aging: Clubs, Meals-on-Wheels, Home-Help Services. In *Growing Old: Problems of Old Age in the Australian Community,* edited by Stoller, A. Melbourne, F. W. Cheshire, Publisher, First Edition, 1960.

48. Donnelly, J.: Psychiatric therapy in the geriatric patient. *J. Am. Geriatrics Soc., 2*:665, 1954.

49. Dovenmuehle, R. H.; Newman, E. G. and Busse, E. W.: Physical problems of psychiatrically hospitalized elderly persons. *J. Am. Geriatrics Soc., VIII*:11, 1960.

50. Dreikurs, R.: The psychological and philosophical significance of rhythm. *Bulletin of N.A.M.T., X*:4, 1961.

51. Ebaugh, F. G.: Age introduces stress into the family. *Geriatrics,* 2-146, 1956.

52. Emery, M.: Occupational Therapy. In Lawton, G.: *New Goals for Old Age.* New York, Columbia Univ. Press, 1945.

53. Federal Council on Aging: Programs, Resources for Older People. Report to the President. Washington, D. C., Government Printing Office, 1959.

54. Fenichel, O.: *The Psychoanalytic Theory of Neurosis.* New York, Norton, 1945.

55. Ferderber, M. B.: Aspects of rehabilitation of the aged. *J.A.M.A., 162*:11, 1956.

56. Ferguson, J. T.: A new therapeutic approach to abnormal behavior in geriatrics. *Geriatrics, 11*:217-219, 1956.

57. Fidler, S. G., and Fidler, J. W.: *Psychiatric Occupational Therapy.* New York, The MacMillen Co., 1954.

58. Freeman, J. T.: History of geriatrics. *Ann. M. Hist., 10*:324, 1938.

59. Freeman, J. T.: The mechanisms of stress and the forces of senescence. *J. Am. Geriatrics Soc.,* 7:71, 1959.
60. Freud, S.: On Psychotherapy. In *Collected Papers, Vol. 1.* London, Hogarth Press, 1924.
61. Freyhan, F. A.: Clinical effectiveness of tofranil in the treatment of depressive psychosis. *Canad. Psychiat.* A. *J.,* 4:Supplement, 586, 597, 1958.
62. Gasster, M.: Clinical experience with L'Glutavite in aged patients with behavior problems and memory defects. *J. Am. Geriatrics Soc., IX*:5, 370, 1961.
63. Gerard, R. W.: Some Aspects of Neural Growth, Regeneration and Function. In *Genetic Neurology,* edited by P. Weiss. Chicago, Univ. of Chicago Press, 1950.
64. Gericke, O. D.; Lobb, L. G.; and Pardoll, D. M.: An evaluation of procaine in geriatric patients in a mental hospital. *J. Clin. Exper. Psychopath.,* 22:1, 18-33, 1961.
65. Gerty, F.: Importance of individualization of treatment in the aging period. *Geriatrics, 12*:123-129, 1957.
66. Geschickter, C. F.: Some Fundamental Aspects of the Aging Process. In V. A. Prospectus, *Research in Aging.* U. S. Govt. Printing Office, Washington, D. C., 1959.
67. Gilbert, J. G.: *Understanding Old Age.* New York, Ronald, 1952.
68. Gitelson, M.: The emotional problems of elderly people. *Geriatrics, 3*:135-150, 1948.
69. Goldfarb, A. I., and Turner, H.: Psychotherapy for aged persons, utilization and effectiveness of 'brief' therapy. *Am. J. Psychiat., 109*:12, 1953.
70. Goldfarb, A. I.: Psychotherapy of aged persons, one aspect of the psychodynamics of the therapeutic situation with aged patients. *Psychoanalyt. Rev., 42*:2, 1955.
71. Goldfarb, A. I.: Psychotherapy of the Aged. The use and value of an adaptational frame of reference. *Psychoanalyt. Rev. 43*: 1, 1958.
72. Goldfarb, A. I.: Prevalence of psychiatric disorders in metropolitan old age and nursing homes. *J. Am. Geriatrics Soc., X*:1, 1962.
73. Grotjahn, M.: Analytic psychotherapy with the elderly. *Psychoanalyt. Rev.,* 42, *4*:419-427, 1955.
74. Grotjahn, M.: Psychoanalytic investigation of a seventy-one year old man with senile dementia. *Psychoanalyt. Quart.,* 9:80-97, 1940.

75. Gumpert, M.: Geriatrics and Social Work. Presented to: Institute on Group Work and Recreation with the Aged, Western Reserve Univ., Cleveland, Ohio, April 16, 1953.
76. Havighurst, R. J.: Successful aging. *Gerontologist, 1*:1, 1961.
77. Hill, B. H.: Here's what recreation can do for geriatric patients. *Geriatrics, 16*:11, 1961.
78. Himwich, H. E.: *Brain Metabolism and Cerebral Disorders.* Baltimore, The Williams and Wilkins Co., 1951.
79. Himwich, H. E.: Wolff, K.; Hunsicker, A. L.; and Himwich, W. A.: Some behavioral effects associated with feeding sodium glutamate to patients with psychiatric disorders. *J. Nerv. & Ment. Dis.*, 121-40-59, 1955.
80. Himwich, H. E., and Himwich, W. A.: Brain Metabolism in Relation to Aging. In *The Neurologic and Psychiatric Aspects of the Aging.* Baltimore, Williams and Wilkins, 1956.
81. Hutchinson, E. D.: The nature of insight. *Psychiatry, Vol. IV*, 1941.
82. Hyde, R. W., and Atwell, C. R.: Evaluating the effectiveness of a psychiatric occupational therapy program. *Am. J. Occup. Therapy*, II, Nov.-Dec., 1948.
83. Jackson, Don D. (Editor): *The Etiology of Schizophrenia.* New York, Basic Books, Inc., 1960.
84. Jelliffee, S. E.: The old age factor in psychoanalytic therapy. *M. J. Rec., 121*:7-12, 1925.
85. Johnson, L. R.: The modern nursing home. Special Geronto-Therapy Issue. Reprinted from Issue of *The New Physician*, July, 1961.
86. Jones, H. E., and Kaplan, O. S.: Psychological Aspects of Mental Disorders in Later Life. In *Mental Disorders in Later Life*, 2nd Edition, edited by O. S. Kaplan. Stanford, Stanford Univ. Press, 1956.
87. Jones, R. T.: Drug Therapy in the Aged. Transactions of the Fifth Research Conference on Cooperative Chemo-Therapy Studies in Psychiatry and Research Approaches to Mental Sickness, June 6-8, 1960, Vol. V, Veterans Adm., Wash. 25., D.C., Dec. 1960.
88. Kaplan, J.: The day center and the day care center. *Geriatrics*, 12, 4, 1957.
89. Kaufman, M. R.: Psychoanalysis in later life depressions. *Psychoanalyt. Quart.* 6:308, 1937.

90. Kaufman, M. R.: Old age and aging. The psychoanalytic point of view. *Am. J. Orthopsychiat.*, 10, 1940.

91. Kety, S. S.: Human Cerebral Blood Flow Oxygen Consumption as Related to Aging. In *The Neurologic and Psychiatric Aspects of the Disorders of Aging.* Baltimore, Williams and Wilkins, 1956.

92. Kety, S. S.: Circulation and metabolism of the human brain in health and disease. *Am. J. Med.*, *8*:205, 1950.

93. Kleemeier, R. W.: The Use and Meaning of Time in Special Settings. In *Aging and Leisure,* R. W. Kleemeier, Editor. New York, Oxford Univ. Press, 1961.

94. Knudson, A. B. C.: Physical medicine and rehabilitation. Application to geriatric problems, *J. Am. Geriatrics Soc.*, *II*:9, 1954.

95. Knudson, A. B. C.: Rehabilitation of the chronically ill in the Veterans Administration. *J.A.M.A.*, *162*:11, 1956.

96. Kolb, L.: The mental hospitalization of the aged. It is overdone? *Am. J. Psychiat.*, *112*:627, 1956.

97. Kubie, S. H., and Landau, G.: *Groupwork with the Aged.* New York, Intern. Univ. Press, Inc., 1953.

98. Kuhlen, R. G.: Aging and Life-Adjustment. In *Handbook of Aging and the Individual,* edited by J. E. Birren. The Univ. of Chicago Press, 1959.

99. Lansing, A. I.: General Physiology. In Cowdry's *Problems of Aging,* Edition 3, edited by A. I. Lansing. Baltimore, Williams and Wilkins, 1952.

100. Leeds, M.: *Aging in Indiana,* The Indiana State Commission on the Aging and Aged, Indianapolis, Ind.

101. Leeds, M.: *Indiana Directory of Philanthropic Homes for the Aged.* Published by Indiana State Commission on the Aging and the Aged, Sept. 1960.

102. Levine, H. A.: Community Programs for the Elderly, The Annals of the American Academy of Political and Social Science, Philadelphia, January 1952.

103. Levy, S.: Pharmacological treatment of aged patients in a state mental hospital. *J.A.M.A*, *155*:1260, 1953.

104. Linden, M. E.: Relationship between social attitudes toward aging and the delinquencies of youth. *Am. J. Psychia.*, *114*: 444, 1957.

105. Linden, M. E.: Group psychotherapy with institutionalized senile women: II. Study in gerontologic human relations. *Internat. J. Group Psychotherapy,* 13, 1953.
106. Linden, M. E.: Architecture for Psychogeriatric Installations. Prepared for the Therapy Session on Geriatric Architecture of the Fifth Mental Hospital Institute, Little Rock, Arkansas, October 19-22, 1953.
107. Linden, M. E.: Transference in gerontologic group psychotherapy, IV. Studies in gerontologic human relations. *Internat. J. Group Psychotherapy,* 5, 1955.
108. Linden, M. E.: Geriatrics. In *The Fields of Group Psychotherapy,* edited by S. R. Slavson. New York, Intern. Univ. Press, Inc., 1956.
109. Marazzi, A. S.: Theories on the Mode of Action of Psychopharmacological Agents. In *Recent Advances in Biological Psychiatry, Vol. 3,* edited by Wortis, J. New York, Grune and Stratton, 1961.
110. Martin, A. R.: The fear of relaxation and leisure. *Am. J. Psychoanalysis, XI*:1, 1951.
111. Masserman, J. H.: Biodynamic Therapy in the Aging. An Integration. In *Progress in Psychotherapy,* edited by Masserman, J. H., and Moreno, J. L. New York, Grune and Stratton, 1957.
112. Meerloo, J. A. M.: Modes of psychotherapy in the aged. *J. Am. Geriatrics Soc. IX*:3, 225, 1961.
113. Meerloo, J. A. M.: Psychotherapy with elderly people. *Geriatrics, 10*:583, 1955.
114. Meerloo, J. A. M.: Transference and Resistance in Geriatric Psychotherapy. *Psychoanalyt. Rev., 42*:72, 1955.
115. Menninger, K.: Abuse of rest in psychiatry. *J.A.M.A., 125*:1087, 1944.
116. Menninger, W. C.: Recreation and mental health. *Recreation,* Nov. 1948.
117. Menninger, W. C.: Psychological aspects of hobbies. *Am. J. Psychiatry, 99*:1, 1942.
118. Menninger, K.: Regulatory Devices of the Ego Under Major Stress. Conference at the Intern. Congress of Psychoanalysis, London, July 28, 1953. In K. Menninger, *A Psychiatrist's World, Vol. II.* New York, The Viking Press, 1959, p. 497.
119. Miles, W. R.: Correlation of reaction and coordination speed with age in adults. *Am. J. Psychol., 43*:377, 1931.

120. Oberndorf, C. P.: Sublimation in occupational therapy. *Occup. Therapy & Rehabilitation, 11*:155, 1932.
121. *Observations on Care of the Aging in Europe.* House Committee Print No. 152. Printed for the use of the Committee on Veterans Affairs, U.S. Govt. Printing Office, Washington, D.C., 1961.
122. Overholzer, W.: Some mental problems of aging and their management. *M. Ann., District of Columbia, 10*:212, 1941.
123. Page, H. F.: Medical Aspects of the Health Care Needs of the Elderly Patient. Proceedings of Institute on Health Care Needs of the Elderly Patient, V.A. Center, Kecoughtan, Va., May 4 and 5, 1961.
124. Polner, W.: Day hospital for geriatric patients. *Geriatrics, 16*:2, 1961
125. Powdermaker, B. F., and Frank, J. D.: *Group Psychotherapy.* Cambridge, Harvard Univ. Press, 1953.
126. Rechtschaffen, A.; Atkinson, S. and Freeman, J. G.: An intensive treatment program for state hospital geriatric patients. *Geriatrics, 9*:28, 1954.
127. Rechtschaffen, A.: Psychotherapy with geriatric patients. A review of the literature. *Gerontol., 14*:1:73, 1959.
128. Riccitelli, M. L., and Pelz, K. S.: Evolution of a modern home and hospital for the care of the aged and infirm. *J. Am. Geriatrics Soc.,* VIII, *4*:284, 1960.
129. Ross, M.: A review of some recent treatment methods for elderly psychiatric patients. *A.M.A. Arch. Gen. Psychiat., 1*:6, 1959.
130. Rudd, T. N.: Preventing senile dementia. The need for a new approach. *J. Am. Geriatrics Soc.* VII, *4*:322, 1959.
131. Schwartz, E. D., and Goodman, J. I.: Group therapy of obesity in elderly diabetics. *Geriatrics, 7*:280, 1952.
132. Seidel, H.; Silver, A. A.; and Nagel, H.: Effects of metrazol and nicotinamide on psychic and mental disorders in the geriatric patients. A preliminary report. *J. Am. Geriatric Soc., 1*: 280, 1953.
133. Settel, E.: Marsilid for elderly persons, *J. Clin. & Exper. Psychopath. and Quart. Rev. Psychiat. & Neurol., 9*:Supplement, 98-104, 1958.
134. Selye, H.: *The Stress of Life.* New York, McGraw-Hill, 1956.
135. Sheldon, H. D.: The Changing Demographic Profile. In *Handbook of Social Gerontology, Societal Aspects of Aging,* edited by C. Tibbitts. The Univ. of Chicago Press, 1960.

136. Shestack, R.: *Handbook of Physical Therapy,* New York, Springer Publishing Co., Inc., 1956.
137. Shock, N. W.: *Trends in Gerontology,* Second Edition. Stanford, Stanford Univ. Press, 1957.
138. Shock, N. W.: Age changes in some physiologic processes. *Geriatrics, 12*:40, 1957.
139. Shock, N. W.: Public Health and the Aging Population. In *Public Health Reports,* U.S. Dept. of Health, Education, and Welfare, 76, *11*:1023, 1961.
140. Shock, N. W.: Panel discussion on concepts of the medical profession in relation to aging. *J. Am. Geriatrics Soc.,* VIII, *8*: 600, 1960.
141. Silver, A.: Group psychotherapy with senile psychotic women. *Geriatrics, 5*:147, 1950.
142. Smigel, J. O.; Serhus, L. N.; and Barmak, S.: Metrazol. Its place in geriatric therapy. *J. M. Soc.,* New Jersey, *50*:248, 1953.
143. Stieglitz, E. J.: Foundation of Geriatric Medicine. In *Geriatric Medicine,* Third Edition, edited by Stieglitz, E. J. Philadelphia, Lippincott, 1954.
144. Stoller, A.: Education for Aging and the Aged. In *Growing Old.* Problems of Old Age In The Australian Community, edited by Stoller, A. Melbourne, F. W. Cheshire, Publisher, 1960.
145. Vickery, F. E.: *San Francisco Senior Center, Annual Report,* 1957-1958.
146. Wayne, G. J.: Psychotherapy in senescence. *Ann. West. Med. & Surg., 6*:88, 1952.
147. Wayne, G. J.: Modified psychoanalytic therapy in senescence. *Psychoanalyt. Rev., 40*:99, 1953.
148. Wechsler, D.: *The Measurement of Adult Intelligence.* Baltimore, Williams and Wilkins, 1951.
149. Weinberg, J.: Psychotherapy of the Aged Person. In *The Neurological and Psychiatric Aspects of the Disorders of Aging,* edited by J. E. Moore, H. H. Merritt, and R. J. Masselink. Baltimore, The Williams and Wilkins Co., 1956.
150. West, W. L.: *Psychiatric occupational therapy: Am. Occup. Therapy* A., New York, 1959.
151. Wolff, K.: Treatment of the geriatric patient in a mental hospital. *J. Am. Geriatrics Soc., 4*:472, 1956.
152. Wolff, K.: Group psychotherapy with geriatric patients in a mental hospital. *J. Am. Geriatrics Soc., 5*:13, 1957.

153. Wolff, K.: Occupational therapy for geriatric patients in a mental hospital: Therapeutic possibilities and limitations. *J. Am. Geriatrics Soc.,* *5*:1019, 1957.
154. Wolff, K.: Psychiatric evaluation of geriatric patients on an outpatient basis: Preliminary study. *J. Am. Geriatrics Soc.,* *6*:760, 1958.
155. Wolff, K.: Active therapy replaces custodial care of geriatric patients in mental hospitals. *Geriatrics,* *13*:174, 1958.
156. Wolff, K.: Psychiatric treatment of the geriatric patient in a psychiatric hospital setting. *Internat. J. Social Psychiat.,* Anniversary Edition, VI, 1 and 2, 1960.
157. Wolff, K.: Group psychotherapy with geriatric patients in a state mental hospital setting. Results of a three-year study. *Group Psychotherapy,* XII, *3*:218, 1959.
158. Wolff, K.: Group psychotherapy with geriatric patients in a Veterans Administration hospital. *Group Psychotherapy,* XIV, *1-2*:85, 1961.
159. Wolff, K.: L'Glutavite, clinical effects on geriatric patients in a psychiatric hospital. *J. Kansas M. Soc.,* LIX, *7*:310, 1958.
160. Wolff, K.: *The Biological, Sociological and Psychological Aspects of Aging.* Springfield, Thomas, 1959.
161. Wolff, K.; Grasberger, J. C.; and Kidorf, I. W.: Nialamide in the treatment of chronic schizophrenia in geriatric patients: A controlled study. *J. Am. Geriatrics Soc.,* X, *2*:148, 1962.
162. Wolff, K., and Klugler, J.: The Use of Novocaine Therapy for Geriatric Patients. Unpublished study.
163. Wortis, J.: Physiological treatment. *Am. J. Psychiat.,* 118, *7*:595, 1962.
164. Wyman, J. F.: Hydrotherapy. In *Medical Physics,* edited by O. Glasser. Chicago, The Year Book Publisher, Inc., 1950.